Public Health and Health Promotion for Nurses
at a Glance

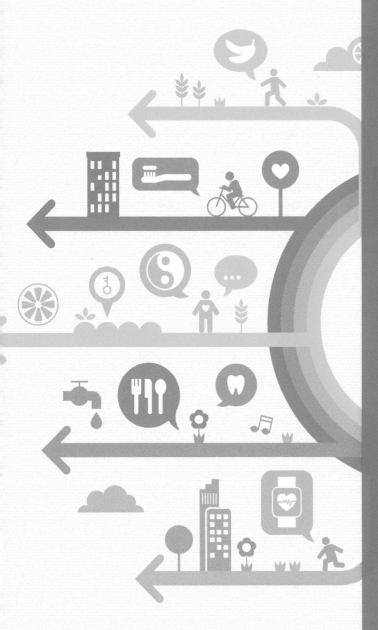

Public Health and Health Promotion for Nurses

at a Glance

Karen Wild
RN, HV, RNT, MA
Formerly of University of Salford
Frederick Road Campus
Salford, UK

Maureen McGrath
Nurse, Health Visitor Community
Practice Teacher, MSc
Formerly of University of Salford
Mary Seacole Building
Frederick Road Campus
Greater Manchester
Salford, UK

WILEY Blackwell

Registered Offices: John Wiley & Sons, Inc., 111 River Street, Hoboken, NJ 07030, USA
                         John Wiley & Sons Ltd, The Atrium, Southern Gate, Chichester,
                         West Sussex, PO19 8SQ, UK

Editorial Office: 9600 Garsington Road, Oxford, OX4 2DQ, UK

For details of our global editorial offices, customer services, and more information about Wiley products visit us at www.wiley.com.

Wiley also publishes its books in a variety of electronic formats and by print-on-demand. Some content that appears in standard print versions of this book may not be available in other formats.

Library of Congress Cataloging-in-Publication Data is available.
Paperback ISBN: 9781119274186

Cover Design: Wiley
Cover Image: © DrAfter123/Getty Images

Set in Minion Pro 9.5/11.5 by Aptara
Printed and bound by CPI Group (UK) Ltd, Croydon, CR0 4YY

10 9 8 7 6 5 4 3 2 1

Karen dedicates this text to her mother, Molly.

*Maureen dedicates this text to her father, Thomas,
who died aged 90 years during its development.*

Contents

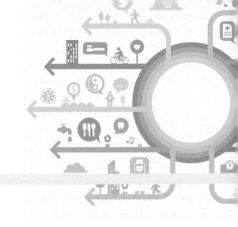

Preface

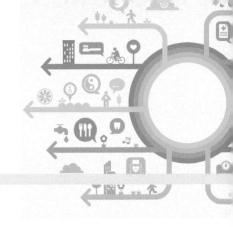

The purpose of this book is to bring together ideas and theories around public health and health promotion in an easily accessed format. It highlights how nurses can work to promote the health of individual patients and communities. There are six units, each with a specific theme designed to link with each other throughout the book.

Unit 1 will consider what public health has to do with nursing. The idea here is to indicate the congruence between the outcomes of public health and the outcomes of nursing.

In Unit 2 the focus moves to health promotion. The message that we want to convey here is that health promotion is not 'an addition' to core nursing work, it is central to compassionate and authentic nursing care. Everything a nurse does has the potential to promote health for a patient.

Hospitals are unhealthy places and we want to encourage readers to think about ways of preventing people either coming into hospital in the first place or returning because of an inability to manage acute illness or a longer term condition. This is the focus of Unit 3.

In Unit 4 we will explore some of the skills – particularly communication skills – used in supporting behaviour change. In this unit we want to challenge the mantra that 'nurses have not got time to "do" health promotion.

The penultimate unit, Unit 5, will look at the skills needed to engage a community in thinking about the factors that impact on their health and about strategies to improve health.

In the final unit, Unit 6, we will share our belief that health promotion is fraught with ethical dilemmas concerning autonomy, beneficence, non-maleficence and justice, and engage the reader in exploring the stewardship approach to the ethics of public health and health promotion.

Karen Wild
Maureen McGrath

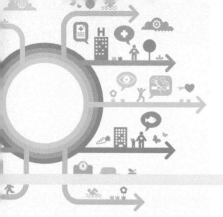

Acknowledgements

Karen would like to acknowledge the support of Gary, David and her mum, Molly, who at the age of 86 is an excellent example of health in later years!

Both authors acknowledge the kind use of resources from Public Health England and NHS publications.

Maureen would like to acknowledge the support and patience of family and friends.

Authors' biographies

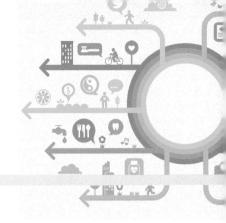

Karen Wild RN, HV, RNT, MA.

Karen's nursing career spans 39 years. She has an established interest in adult and community nursing. Prior to becoming a nurse educator, she worked as a Health Visitor where she gained an interest in public health nursing and family care. As a Senior Lecturer in nursing, she has extended her area of interest into self-awareness and leadership.

Maureen McGrath Nurse, Health Visitor Community Practice Teacher, MSc (retired)

Maureen qualified as a Registered General Nurse in 1977 at Sheffield School of Nursing. She completed Health Visitor training at Sheffield Polytechnic and Community Practice Teacher training at Bolton College. She gained an MSc (Practitioner Research) from Manchester Metropolitan University. Maureen worked as a lecturer at the University of Salford. Her teaching and research interests were related to public health, health promotion and behaviour change. Maureen was Programme Leader for the Post-Graduate MA.

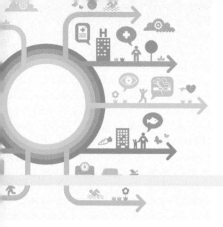

Glossary of terms

BMI: body mass index.

Director of Nursing for Public Health: appointed in 2011 to advise the government on nursing policy and development in relation to public health.

District Nurse: a registered nurse with an extra specialist practitioner qualification.

Domains of health: these include physical, mental, emotional, social, sexual and societal health.

Emotional health: recognition and appropriate expression of feelings, plus the ability to cope with stress.

Epidemiology: analyses the way diseases are spread between populations and the factors that influence their distribution.

Green Book: a resource produced by the Department of Health to aid practitioners who are immunising against infectious diseases.

Health education: has a focus mainly on giving information to change people's health behaviour, e.g. propaganda and instruction.

Health inequalities: an analysis of the gap or gradient in health between population groups that can usually be measured by a number of social characteristics.

Health promotion: involves empowerment of individuals and seeks to alter attitudes in order that people might change their health behaviours.

Health protection: teams work alongside the NHS to provide information, advice and expertise, as well as emergency response during disease outbreaks.

Health surveillance: the continuous, systematic collection, analysis and interpretation of health-related data needed for the planning, implementation and evaluation of public health practice.

Health Visitor: a qualified nurse who has undergone extra education on the recognised Health Visitor programme of study.

Marmot Review: into health equity and inequality acknowledges that health outcomes are poorer in societies in which inequalities exist (socioeconomic inequalities, inequality of opportunity, inequality of provision of education, housing, green spaces, etc.).

Mental health: clear and coherent thinking; here cognitive abilities can be measured, for example in children's developmental assessment and in the elderly who may be suffering from dementia.

Morbidity: the incidence of illness within the population.

Mortality: the incidence of death by cause within the population.

Motivational interviewing: a method of motivating individuals to think about their health behaviour.

NICE (National Institute for Health and Care Excellence): provides national guidance for the prevention and treatment of major illnesses.

Physical health: how your body functions, which can often be in terms of measuring physical parameters, for example blood pressure monitoring, body mass index measurement, assessment of motor development in children.

Primary care nursing: focused in the community setting to support all people who need nursing support in their home environment.

Primary prevention: geared towards preventing the onset of disease.

Public health: an overarching term that covers aspects of health promotion and disease prevention.

Public Health England: an executive agency of the Department of Health.

School Nurse: a registered nurse who specialises in supporting the health and wellbeing of school-aged children. May have an extra qualification as a Specialist Community Public Health Nurse.

Secondary prevention: identifies individuals or groups at risk of disease with the aim of detecting and curing illnesses before they cause irreversible ill health.

Sexual health: the acceptance and ability to achieve a satisfactory expression of one's sexuality.

Social health: the ability to make and maintain relationships with others.

Societal health: being valued within society, regardless of religion, race, age, gender, etc.

Specialist Community Public Health Nurse: a registered nurse who has undergone specialist postqualification education in community public health nursing.

Spiritual health: being at peace with oneself through a system of beliefs.

Tertiary prevention: aims to minimise or reduce the progression of an already established disease.

What has public health to do with nursing?

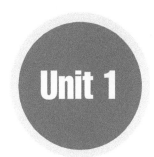

Unit 1

Chapters

Thinking points for NMC Revalidation

Once you have completed Unit 1 you will have gained an insight into why public health nursing is such an important part of the NMC competencies. How does it relate to the work that you carry out in practice?

1 What is public health and why is it relevant to nursing?

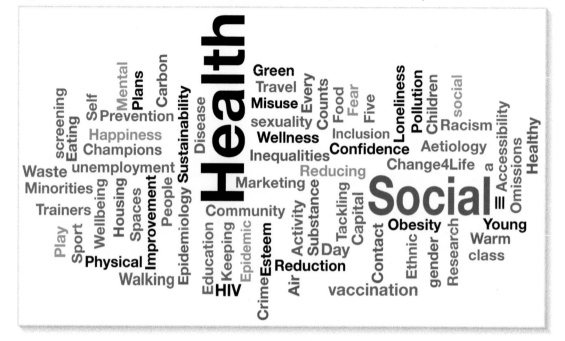

Figure 1.1.1 What is public health? Source: Adapted from Public Health Hub, Sheffield Hallam University.

Table 1.1.1 Public health outcomes. Source: Department of Health (2012). Licensed under Open Government Licence v3.0. http://www.nationalarchives.gov.uk/doc/open-government-licence/version/3/.

Domain 2: Health improvement	Domain 4: Health care, public health and preventing premature mortality
Objective: Help people to live healthy lifestyles, make healthy choices and reduce health inequalities	**Objective:** Reduce numbers of people with preventable long-term ill health and reduce numbers of people dying prematurely, while reducing the gap between communities

Box 1.1.1 Extracts from the Standards for Competence for Registered Nurses. Source: Nursing and Midwifery Council (2015). http://www.nmc.org.uk/globalassets/sitedocuments/standards/nmc-standards-for-competence-for-registered-nurses.pdf.

All nurses must:

- act on their understanding of how people's lifestyles, environments and where care is delivered, influence their health and wellbeing
- seek out every opportunity to promote health and prevent illness
- understand public health principles, priorities and practice in order to recognise and respond to the major causes and social determinants of health, illness and health inequalities

Public Health and Health Promotion for Nurses at a Glance, First Edition. Karen Wild and Maureen McGrath.
© 2019 John Wiley & Sons Ltd. Published 2019 by John Wiley & Sons Ltd.

Public health: definition

A number of definitions exist – probably the best is the one used by Acheson (1988):

the science and art of preventing disease, prolonging life, and promoting health through the organised efforts of society

Public health is generally thought of as those strategies that impact on population health such as screening programmes and vaccination programmes, but it is about much more than that (Figure 1.1.1).

The definition that is posted on the current GOV.UK Public Health page is:

Public health is about helping people to stay healthy, and protecting them from threats to their health. The government wants everyone to be able to make healthier choices, regardless of their circumstances, and to minimise the risk and impact of illness.

www.gov.uk/government/topics/public-health

The approach to public health of the current administration has been to place an emphasis on health improvement and prevention of ill health, largely through support for changing health behaviours, and this has been at the centre of its strategy for health in England (Department of Health, 2010), which has the overall aim of

helping people live longer, healthier and more fulfilling lives; and improving the health of the poorest, fastest. … tackling the wider social determinants of health. This new approach will aim to build people's self-esteem, confidence and resilience right from infancy.

Department of Health, 2010, p. 4

The strategy is concerned with addressing the inequalities in health that were recognised in the Marmot Review (Marmot, 2010) into health equity and inequality. This review acknowledges that health outcomes are poorer in societies in which inequalities exist (socioeconomic inequalities, inequality of opportunity, inequality of provision of education, housing, green spaces. etc.).

For those of you interested in the link between wealth inequalities and health inequalities, you may wish to access the Equality Trust site (http://www.equalitytrust.org.uk/) and also a book, *The Spirit Level* (Wilkinson and Pickett, 2009).

In England there is as yet little evidence that the gap between the health (measured in terms of mortality and morbidity) of the poorest and the richest is narrowing. It is also the case that for many health indicators England fares worse than other developed countries. For example, although mortality rates for cardiovascular disease (CVD) have fallen they are still high compared with other developed countries (only Ireland and Finland have higher rates). Death rates due to CVD are six times higher in people from lower socioeconomic groups when compared with those from higher socioeconomic groups. Most premature deaths from CVD are preventable and the government's strategy has been built on a belief that this is also the case for many other conditions – some cancers, respiratory diseases (particularly chronic obstructive pulmonary disease, or COPD), some mental health conditions, overweight and obesity. There has been a welcome acknowledgement of the impact of mental health and wellbeing on physical health, and vice versa.

Public health: relevance to nursing

So what does public health have to do with nursing? Most people spend a relatively small proportion of their overall lifespan in contact with nurses and in the main that contact occurs at a time of acute ill health when the emphasis is on 'getting better' or 'recovery'. There is a recognition that nurses are ideally placed to support people to make healthier choices because of the nature of the therapeutic relationship that develops between a nurse and a patient/client/family and because that relationship develops at a time when people are facing their vulnerabilities to illness and other threats to their health.

The current Nursing and Midwifery Council (NMC) competency standards for registered nurses (Nursing and Midwifery Council, 2015) indicate the requirement for nurses to understand public health principles and be able to respond appropriately to support people in managing the many different factors that impact on health and wellbeing (Box 1.1.1). **All** nurses are required to be able to recognise the existence of and deterioration in mental health and wellbeing – this is of particular relevance when a nurse is engaging someone in behaviour change. There is also the requirement to recognise that different stages in people's lives represent different challenges and vulnerabilities to ill health. They also represent different opportunities to improve health and wellbeing as nurses engage with patients in different contexts.

The Public Health Outcomes Framework 2013–2016 (Department of Health, 2012) has two domains that directly relate to the work that nurses engage in with patients (Table 1.1.1). The need for a focus on prevention of ill health is also outlined in the multi-agency five-year plan drawn together by the Chief Executive of NHS England, Simon Stevens, in order to ensure the sustainability of the National Health Service (NHS) as we know it.

It is important to note that the responsibility for public health – in the sense of improving health and wellbeing – was transferred from health trusts to local authorities following the Health and Social Care Act 2012. In July 2015 the Conservative government announced a 6.2% reduction in the funds that would be made available to local authorities for spending on public health. It is therefore imperative that nurses engage in every opportunity afforded to them to improve the health and wellbeing of patients/clients/families.

2 Some historical points of public health

Figure 1.2.3 Public Health Act 1848.
Source: http://www.nationalarchives.gov.uk/education/victorianbritain/healthy/source6f.htm. Licensed under Open Government Licence v3.0, http://www.nationalarchives.gov.uk/doc/open-government-licence/version/3/.

Figure 1.2.1 Edwin Chadwick.

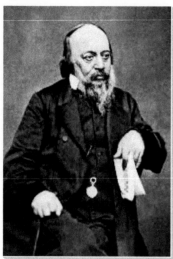

Figure 1.2.2 Victorian industrial housing.

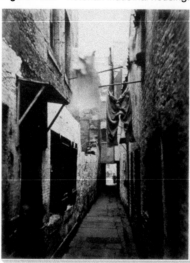

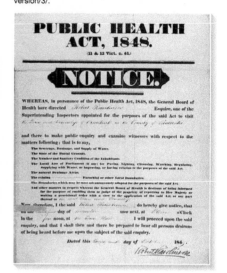

Figure 1.2.4 The incidence of death from pertussis in the general population and in infants within the twentieth century in the UK. Source: National Archives. Licensed under Open Government Licence v3.0. http://www.nationalarchives.gov.uk/doc/open-government-licence/version/.

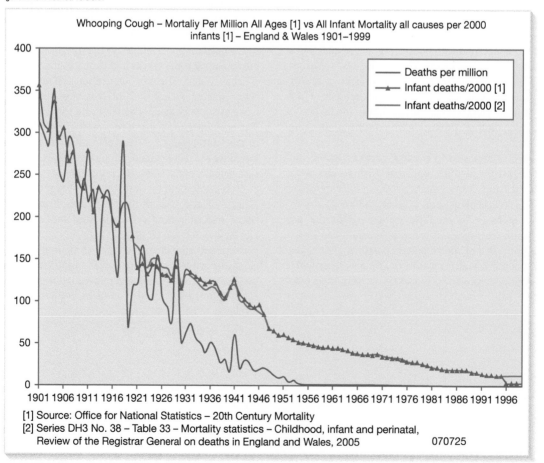

[1] Source: Office for National Statistics – 20th Century Mortality
[2] Series DH3 No. 38 – Table 33 – Mortality statistics – Childhood, infant and perinatal, Review of the Registrar General on deaths in England and Wales, 2005   070725

Public Health and Health Promotion for Nurses at a Glance, First Edition. Karen Wild and Maureen McGrath.
© 2019 John Wiley & Sons Ltd. Published 2019 by John Wiley & Sons Ltd.

Our understanding of contemporary public health is enhanced by viewing its historical context, and by building on our knowledge of the past it can be argued that we are better placed to appreciate current intervention within public health.

The convention of public health and people's comprehension of the idea dates as early as pre-Christian times. Rosen (1993; cited in Costello and Haggart, 2003) identifies five important historical periods: the Graeco-Romans with an emphasis on water and sanitation; the medieval focus on endemics; the Enlightenment and a focus on disease prevalence; the industrial focus on working conditions; and a modern era with a focus on bacteriology and virology.

Our forefathers were of the notion that the environment had a huge influence on health and disease, and as such the quality or inadequacy of the air was important. Better to live in airy, well-ventilated places than to reside in the toxic environment of rotting debris, or humid environments. The agricultural revolution saw the expansion of the population, and consequently the development of settlements, villages and towns. The summer months were synonymous with the putrefaction of debris, when the smell was at its worse and the presence of disease was acutely observed. Belief systems supported this view, and the use of aromatic oils, herbs and flowers to deodorise and 'cleanse' the environment was popular. The balance of bodily humours was thought to enhance health, with blood, phlegm, yellow and black bile in harmony with the elements of air, fire, earth and water, and the qualities of wet, dry, hot and cold. In contemporary society, there is still the notion of exposure to cold and wet as being the cause of colds and influenza.

Early religious control and the interpretation of sickness and ill health related to devil worship or diabolism, which enhanced the moral stance of communities, and as a consequence, victim blaming was rife. Fear and superstition went hand in hand with ignorance and a lack of education. At the time of the Enlightenment, the period between 1700 and 1850, a more scientific approach began to emerge, as social values and democracy became key themes. This coupled with the effects of industrialisation and an explosion of development in our towns and cities sparked a public and political response. So-called progress brought with it a set of health problems that were endemic in Europe and America.

In the early 1800s Jeremy Bentham and his band of theoretical radicals developed the philosophy of utilitarianism, which provided a benchmark for health policy and wider social policy. Philanthropists expressed concern about the health and welfare of their workers, and housing and communities with schools and hospitals emerged. In addition, good health amongst workers supported the capitalist production and profits.

In a Viennese hospital in the 1840s, Ignaz Semmelweis observed the incidence of postpartum sepsis. Two maternity wards existed, one run exclusively by midwives, and the other used as a training facility for medical students. The students had often attended births straight from the dissecting room where they had been working on corpses with their bare hands. Sepsis was observed to be much more prevalent in the medical student ward. Semmelweis made the assumption that contagion was carried on the hands; medical students were instructed to wash hands in chlorinated lime water and rates of infection dramatically reduced.

John Snow is thought to be the father of epidemiology as a result of his systematic studies over decades looking into the spread of cholera in London. For a really insightful overview of his work, together with that of Reverend Johnston, have a look at author Steven Johnson discussing a cholera outbreak in Victorian London (https://www.youtube.com/watch?v=3P8shnNEXb4). Cholera continues to be a worldwide problem today, and was epidemic following the Haiti earthquake in 2010.

Alongside scientific awareness and the social value of intelligence, was the recognition that poor health fell disproportionately upon the poorer members of society. The correlation between poverty and mortality rates has persisted for centuries as a powerful predictor of health. Figure 1.2.1 shows Sir Edwin Chadwick, who in 1842 proved that life expectancy was much lower in towns than in the countryside. He was a key proponent of the 'sanitary idea' and was instrumental in the development of central public health administration. In the UK, particularly in the industrial north, housing became cramped, with narrow streets and back-to-back houses with shared courtyards and shared outside toilets; in 1850s Manchester 250 people had to share two 'privies' (Figure 1.2.2). In 1848, the Public Health Act was passed by Robert Peel's government, establishing a Central Board of Health responsible for water supply and drainage (Figure 1.2.3). This was subsequently revised in 1858 and the Central Board abolished to devolve responsibility to Local Boards to reform conditions and focus on the prevention of ill health.

In 1853 Louis Pasteur studied the fermentation of beer and its links with microbes. He subsequently developed the process of milk pasteurisation, and identified aerobic and anaerobic microorganisms. Together with Jenner's work on smallpox vaccines, he developed vaccines for human use (rabies) and for sheep (anthrax) and poultry (cholera).

At the turn of the twentieth century, infectious diseases such as measles, diphtheria, smallpox and pertussis (or whooping cough) were widely prevalent, and the incidence of mortality from such infections was high. The development and use of vaccines has dramatically influenced the reduction of morbidity and mortality from these diseases (Figure 1.2.4) and even enabled the eradication worldwide of smallpox.

Other achievements in public health in the twentieth century include improvements in working conditions, health and safety legislation, and the introduction of legislation to reduce pollutants. Food safety to improve sanitation and hygiene practices alongside fluoridation of water has also contributed to enhanced health. Family planning and the improvements in maternal and child health have seen a 90% overall reduction in infant mortality, and a 99% reduction of maternal mortality.

Improvements in standards of living, diet, access to health care, and the surveillance and monitoring of disease have positively enhanced public health and the outcomes of health to population groups.

Social control is seen as the mechanism by which public health has been organised over the last 200 years or so. Contemporary public health draws from these historical achievements. New public health measures are suggestive of increased surveillance, and many commentators have described the 'nannying' effect of moral regulation on the population. The current UK government advocates policies that recommend preventive strategies, and promotes authority based on surveillance, screening and measuring targets, a method commonly ascribed to a medical model of health. These themes will be developed in further chapters.

3 Determinants of health

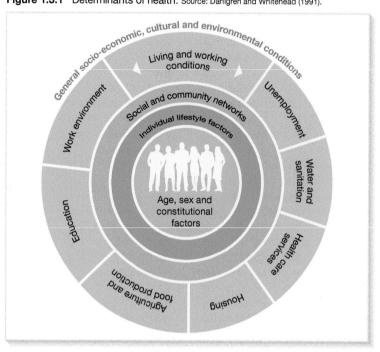

Figure 1.3.1 Determinants of health. Source: Dahlgren and Whitehead (1991).

General socio-economic, cultural and environmental conditions

Living and working conditions

Unemployment

Work environment

Social and community networks

Individual lifestyle factors

Water and sanitation

Education

Age, sex and constitutional factors

Health care services

Agriculture and food production

Housing

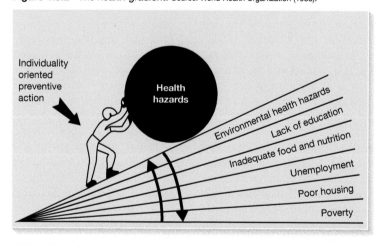

Figure 1.3.2 The health gradient. Source: World Health Organization (1988).

Individuality oriented preventive action

Health hazards

Environmental health hazards

Lack of education

Inadequate food and nutrition

Unemployment

Poor housing

Poverty

Health

Health can be measured using any number of health indicators, some examples of these are:

- Blood pressure
- Cholesterol ratio
- Weekly alcohol intake
- Body Mass Index (BMI)
- Prevalence of dental caries
- Incidence and prevalence of childhood accidents
- Sense of wellbeing
- Hospital admissions for a particular disease/condition.

The Office for National Statistics (http://www.ons.gov.uk/) collects and publishes data on these and many more different health indicators along with changes and trends that occur over time. These measures might be considered to be risk factors for ill health and they are often the factors that nurses are involved in assessing and measuring for patients they meet in primary, secondary or tertiary health settings. It is also important for nurses to be aware of the determinants of health.

Determinants of health

Determinants of health are those factors that influence the incidence and prevalence of risk factors and provide some understanding of why particular risk factors develop in individuals, communities and populations. Determinants of health can be thought of as all of those factors that impact negatively or positively on the health of individuals, families and communities (Figures 1.3.1 and 1.3.2). There is evidence that the broader determinants of health (particularly factors such as educational achievement, employment status and income) have a greater impact on an individual's or a population's experience of health than health care services (Bunker et al., 1995; McGinnis et al., 2002; Marmot, 2010; Canadian Institute of Health Research, quoted in Kuznetsova, 2012).

Individual demographics and genotype, lifestyle, social capital and the socio-political determinants of health (access to education, housing, health and social care services, employment, healthy work environment, healthy food) all interact with each other to influence health experience in different ways for different individuals and in different ways for any one individual at different stages of their life.

Examples

A Take the example of the demographic of age. People are vulnerable to different influences on health at different points in the life course, with the very young and the very old being vulnerable to the greatest impact of a number of determinants. The very young have an immature immune system in response to some infectious illnesses, whereas the very old have an immune system that will not always produce an adequate response to some infectious illnesses. If this reduced immune response is combined with other negative influences on health such as a cold, damp environment, lack of social contact, inadequate nutrition and either a lack of knowledge about or a lack of resources to deal with symptoms of an infectious illness then the consequences may be very serious

B The impact of lifestyle will be much more serious for some people than others – again because of the confounding influence of other determinants of health. A person who has a sedentary lifestyle and who also has a diet high in fats and refined sugars may well begin to display symptoms such as overweight, high blood pressure and high cholesterol ratio that suggest they are at risk of a serious cardiovascular illness, such as coronary heart disease, stroke or type 2 diabetes. If someone in this position also has a familial genetic predisposition to early onset hypertension, coronary heart disease or stroke then the consequences of their lifestyle may be significantly more serious than for someone who does not have this sort of family history.

What does this mean for nurses?

Nurses therefore need to be aware of the contexts within which people live their lives and to understand that individuals may have limited control over many of the determinants that influence their health and may have limitations on their choices in relation to health behaviours. This awareness needs to influence the support and guidance that nurses deliver to patients.

Provision of written health education material is only useful if the patient is able to read and understand it and has the cognitive and economic resources to take advantage of the information.

Patients may struggle to follow a complex medication regime if their family circumstances are chaotic, or if they are socially isolated.

People might find attendance at follow-up appointments difficult if given a written appointment card months in advance with no reminder, or if their mobility is poor and/or they do not have/cannot afford transport.

Advice to change a health behaviour (diet/exercise/smoking) will be difficult in the absence of ongoing encouragement/support or in an environment that encourages negative health behaviours.

Units 2 and 4 will address these issues further.

Health improvement and the role of the nurse

Table 1.4.1 The two domains. Source: Department of Health (2012).

Domain 2: Health improvement	Domain 4: Health care, public health and preventing premature mortality
Objective: Help people to live healthy lifestyles, make healthy choices and reduce health inequalities	**Objective:** Reduce numbers of people with preventable long-term ill health and reduce numbers of people dying prematurely, while reducing the gap between communities.

Table 1.4.2 Obesity: identification, assessment and management. Source: NICE (2014).

BMI classification	Waist circumference		
	Low	High	Very high
Overweight	No increased risk	Increased risk	High risk
Obesity 1	Increased risk	High risk	Very high risk

For men, waist circumference of less than 94 cm is low, 94–102 cm is high and more than 102 cm is very high.
For women, waist circumference of less than 80 cm is low, 80–88 cm is high and more than 88 cm is very high.

Box 1.4.1 Case study: Colin.

Colin is a 57-year-old painter and decorator who is admitted for routine surgery for inguinal hernia repair. As part of his preoperative assessment you first review his records. He has a recent history of hypertension, which has been monitored and treated by his GP. On first meeting with Colin you find him to be calm and receptive, and as you assess his baseline observations, he reveals to you how proud he is of his management and recording of his own blood pressure measurement. You strike up a conversation about his medication, and soon get the impression that Colin is highly motivated to engage in his treatment. Further assessment reveals that Colin has an above-normal waist circumference of 110 cm and a BMI of 38.4. This puts him in the high-risk category in terms of obesity.

Box 1.4.2 Case study: Colin – brief intervention.

- Assess Colin's view of his weight and the diagnosis, and possible health-related behaviour behind his weight gain.
- Explore Colin's eating patterns and physical activity levels.
- Explore any beliefs that Colin may have about eating, physical activity and weight gain that are unhelpful if he wants to lose weight.
- Be aware that people from certain ethnic and socioeconomic backgrounds may be at greater risk of obesity, and may have different beliefs about what is a healthy weight and different attitudes towards weight management.
- Find out what Colin has already tried and how successful this has been, and what he learned from the experience.
- Assess Colin's readiness to adopt changes.
- Assess Colin's confidence in making changes.

Adapted from 'Base assessment of the health risks associated with being overweight or obese in adults on BMI and waist circumference' (NICE, 2006).

Nursing has faced a number of challenges over the last decade – not least of which has been a number of reports that have been critical of the care that nurses provide to patients in the acute setting (Frances Report, Keogh Report, Cavendish Report, Berwick Report, Clwyd-Hart Report – all published in 2013). The Frances Report in particular was critical of the cultures that had developed in some areas that allowed ways of working that were totally lacking in compassion to become the norm. The report also acknowledged the oppressive conditions that some staff were working under and while not absolving anyone of the responsibility to provide excellent care there was a clear recognition of a link between an undervalued and overworked workforce and poor patient care.

In 2012 a new vision and strategy for nursing was published by the NHS Commissioning Board and the Department of Health that introduced the idea of the six fundamental values that should underpin every engagement with patients – the 6Cs. Hospital trusts have embraced the idea of this strategy without necessarily creating an environment or culture in which it might be a reality. There is also a growing body of evidence that suggests that most nurses feel their work environment to be very pressured and that they have a sense of being undervalued (Ball et al., 2013; Ford, 2014).

Into this mix the Department of Health and Public Health England (2013) have added yet another document that details the three levels of public health that nurses and midwives should be involved with – individual, community and population levels. Rather than being yet another unrealistic meaningless task to 'tick off', health promotion is something that nurses can do – and no doubt already do – with many of the patients that they engage with and is something that can make a real difference to the lives of individuals.

The Public Health Outcomes Framework 2013–2016 (Department of Health, 2012) has two domains that directly relate to the work that nurses engage in with patients. Figure 1.4.1 shows the two domains.

The need for a focus on prevention of ill health is also outlined in the multi-agency five-year plan (NHS England et al., 2014) drawn together by the Chief Executive of NHS England, Simon Stevens, in order to ensure the sustainability of the NHS as we know it. Public Health England, in conjunction with the Department of Health, is working on recommendations to make every contact count across all pathways (NHS Commissioning Board and Department of Health, 2012). The importance of 'making every contact count' and developing the skills to support this is highlighted in a range of reports and strategies. Nurses should 'be able to look to clinical leadership for strong direction about how to make every contact count' (Department of Health 2012, p. 10). Resources and tools have been developed to support organisations to do this systematically. The Royal College of Nursing (RCN) view is that 'a new approach should be adopted across the nursing team to ensure all nurses have an increased and more explicit role in public health and sustainable health' (Royal College of Nursing, 2012, p. 9).

In practice this requires the nurse to be skilled in the assessment of individual risks and associated health behaviour; understand the varied models of health; be skilled in supporting and sustaining choices in health-related behaviours; have skills in and provide opportunities for motivational interviewing; and support and develop goals for individuals to promote health and wellbeing. In the case study (Box 1.4.1) Colin is admitted for routine surgery. During the initial assessment, the nurse identifies Colin's risk factor associated with obesity (Figure 1.4.2).

Box 1.4.2 is adapted from NICE guidelines, and intervention in this scenario can be described as brief, where the nurse enquires about behaviour and associated risk factors.

Brief interventions can and do take place in any setting as part of the general communication that nurses have with individuals in their care. Opportunistically this brief intervention can be identified with something as casual as a remark or gesture, a direct request or negative behaviour.

A recognised strategy for being able to deliver structured information and support in a short time is that of a Brief Intervention (Miller and Rollnick, 2002; NICE, 2006; World Health Organization, 2010; National Obesity Observatory, 2011). A Brief Intervention consists of:
• Opportunistic advice, discussion, negotiation or encouragement
• Usually short, 5–15 minutes in length (sometimes with one brief follow-up contact)
• Structured
• Uses skills of motivational interviewing.

An awareness of behaviour theories and the way that they impact on health is an important component of nursing care, and significant in the way nurses engage in health improvement. Subsequent chapters within this text will explore and seek to explain why certain health behaviours and attitudes to health can make patients and individuals behave in certain ways. Good communication and good listening skills come to the fore, and motivational interviewing requires additional skills of empathy and the ability to assess behaviours and to deliver appropriate health improvement interventions.

5 What people think about public health

Figure 1.5.1 Public health concerns. Source: PHE (2014). Licensed under Open Government Licence v3.0., http://www.nationalarchives.gov.uk/doc/open-government-licence/version/3/.

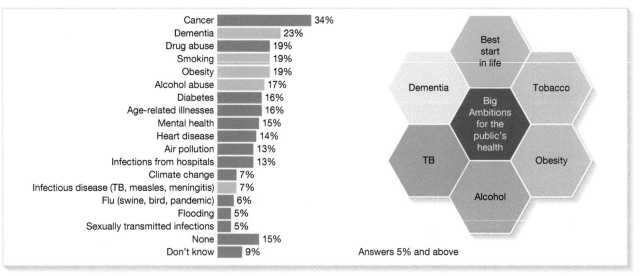

Figure 1.5.2 Over 40s health checks. Source: National Health Service. Licensed under Open Government Licence v3.0., http://www.nationalarchives.gov.uk/doc/open-government-licence/version/3/.

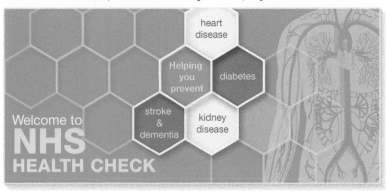

People's perceptions of public health have been recently captured by the British Medical Association (BMA), who conducted a survey to question people's perceptions of the NHS (BMA, 2016). The overwhelming response was in relation to budget cuts to public health funding, with 75% saying they are concerned about cuts to local authority public health budgets. In 2014, the Department of Health reported that three in five people (60%) agree that 'the Government is doing more these days to help people live healthier lives'. This is a slight improvement on the perceptions of the public a decade earlier. In 2006 56% agreed that this was the case. However, this still leaves over one-third of people (35%) disagreeing that the government is doing more to encourage healthier lifestyles.

But what about the public's perception of what public health actually is? Public Health England (PHE, 2014) conducted a public awareness and opinion survey to consider:

- Public health concerns
- Awareness and knowledge of PHE and its role
- Levels of public confidence and trust in PHE.

When people were asked 'Which, if any, public health issues are you concerned about?' 34% said 'cancer' and 23% said 'dementia'. Smaller numbers (only 7%) appeared concerned about infectious diseases. Lifestyle-associated health issues of smoking and obesity accounted for 19% of those concerned. Interestingly, 15% of the respondents said that they were concerned about mental health issues (Figure 1.5.1). MIND reports an increasing awareness amongst the public of mental health issues – this is an upward positive trend.

In the 'winter wave' of the Public Perceptions of the NHS and Social Care Tracker Survey (Department of Health, 2013), when people were asked: 'Who or which organisation, if any, would you contact if you wished to get information on how to stay healthy? This could be advice on how to quit smoking, drink less alcohol, do more exercise, eat more healthily etc', 57% said that they would contact the doctor, GP or nurse. The analysis suggests that most people continue to use traditional methods of communication to consult their GP, with the majority consulting their GP face-to-face. However, there has been a slow but steady increase in the proportion of people contacting NHS services in new ways. In particular, increasing numbers have received text reminders about appointments and have used the

Public Health and Health Promotion for Nurses at a Glance, First Edition. Karen Wild and Maureen McGrath.
© 2019 John Wiley & Sons Ltd. Published 2019 by John Wiley & Sons Ltd.

Figure 1.5.3 Shared decision-making in the NHS. Source: Department of Health. Licensed under Open Government Licence v3.0., http://www.nationalarchives.gov.uk/doc/open-government-licence/version/3/.

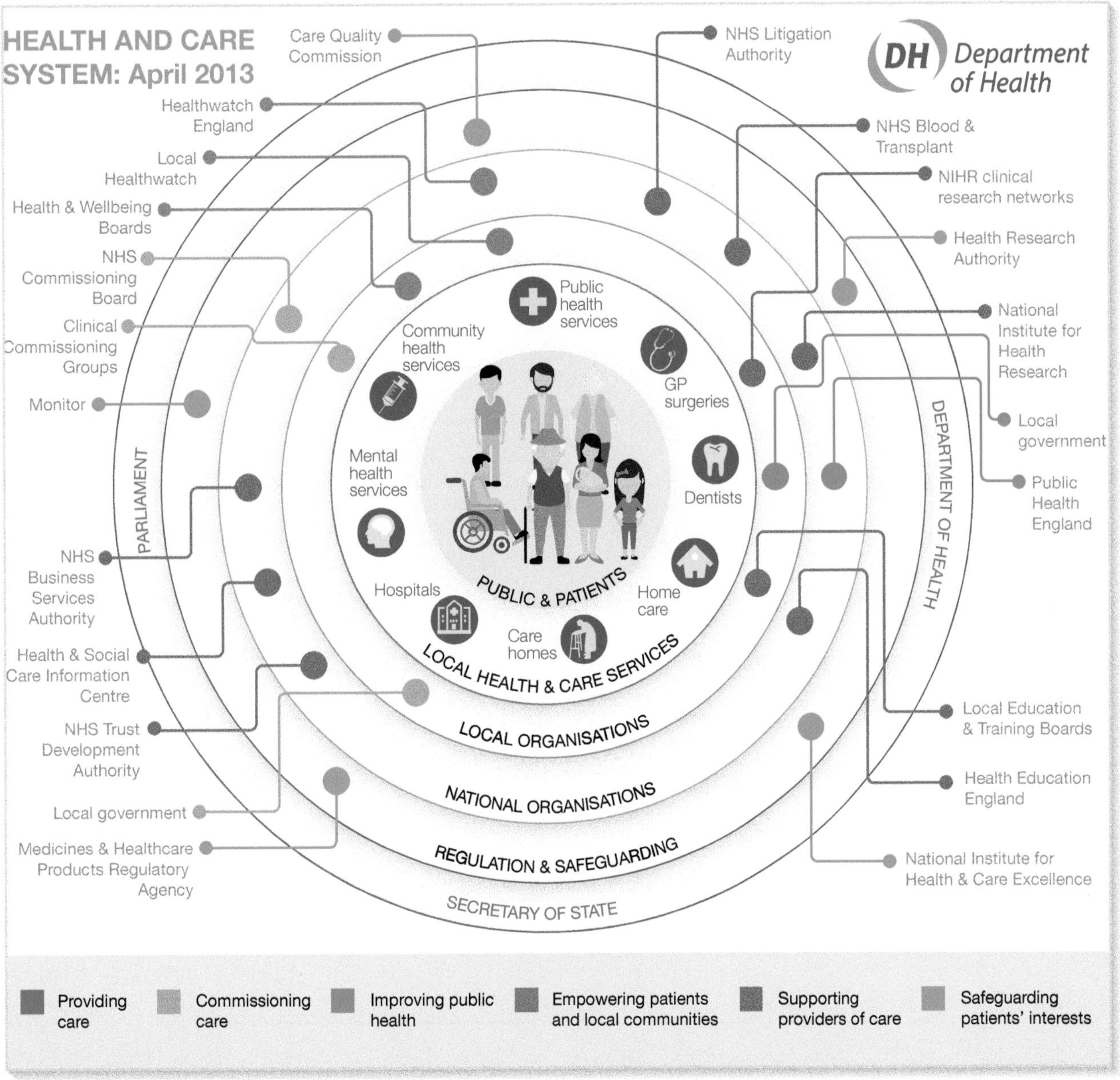

HEALTH AND CARE SYSTEM: April 2013

DH Department of Health

Care Quality Commission
NHS Litigation Authority
Healthwatch England
NHS Blood & Transplant
Local Healthwatch
NIHR clinical research networks
Health & Wellbeing Boards
Health Research Authority
NHS Commissioning Board
National Institute for Health Research
Clinical Commissioning Groups
Local government
Monitor
Public Health England
NHS Business Services Authority
Health & Social Care Information Centre
NHS Trust Development Authority
Local Education & Training Boards
Local government
Health Education England
Medicines & Healthcare Products Regulatory Agency
National Institute for Health & Care Excellence

PARLIAMENT
DEPARTMENT OF HEALTH

Public health services
Community health services
GP surgeries
Mental health services
Dentists
Hospitals
PUBLIC & PATIENTS
Home care
Care homes

LOCAL HEALTH & CARE SERVICES
LOCAL ORGANISATIONS
NATIONAL ORGANISATIONS
REGULATION & SAFEGUARDING
SECRETARY OF STATE

Providing care
Commissioning care
Improving public health
Empowering patients and local communities
Supporting providers of care
Safeguarding patients' interests

NHS 111 service. The appetite for such new methods is growing, with increasing numbers of people keen to be able to book GP appointments online (Department of Health, 2013).

Efforts to raise public awareness of all causes of mortality are promoted by the government and the independent sector. Examples include healthy lifestyles and dementia awareness. Moves to introduce dementia into school curriculums coincide with the news that dementia has taken over as the biggest cause of death in the UK. New figures from the Office for National Statistics (ONS) have shown that dementia and Alzheimer's disease are now the leading cause of death in England and Wales. This replaces ischaemic heart disease as the leading cause of death and is related to an ageing population as well as better dementia diagnosis rates. A way of promoting public health awareness has been introduced into health promotion activities within primary health care. People over the age of 40 in England are to be given more information about dementia to help improve early diagnosis of the condition. During their free NHS health check, patients will be told when they should report memory problems to their GP (Figure 1.5.2).

Public health awareness can be significantly triggered by the media, and TV portrayals of characters on 'soap' programmes and

high-profile individuals can significantly influence public attitudes towards health. MIND and the ITV show Loose Women launched the 'Lighten the Load' campaign, which recognises heroes in everyday life who support those with mental health problems. The campaign challenges the stigma of mental health by engaging with and encouraging open discussion around a variety of mental health issues, allowing people to talk and share their experiences. Topics such as: how to cope after suicide in the family; postnatal depression; depression after a relationship breakup; and spotting signs of anxiety in children are openly shared (http://www.mind.org.uk/news-campaigns/mind-media-awards).

In April 2012 the government set out its model of shared governance, putting the public and patients at the heart of decision making creating a 'no decision about me, without me' ambition (Figure 1.5.3). This gives individuals greater involvement in their own care and a greater say (Department of Health, 2012). The assumption here is that individuals are seen as consumers of care and as such have the right to choose. With consumerism comes a shift of power between professional and patients, with opportunities for shared collaboration in the development and provision of support and care.

6 How public health is measured: epidemiology

Figure 1.6.1 The complexity of epidemiology.

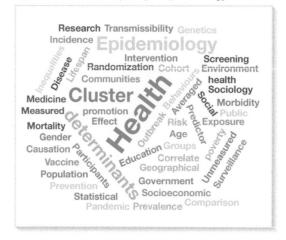

Figure 1.6.2 Cohort life expectancy at birth, UK (1980–2017). Source: Office of National Statistics. Licensed under Open Government Licence v3.0,http://www.nationalarchives.gov.uk/doc/open-government-licence/version/3/.

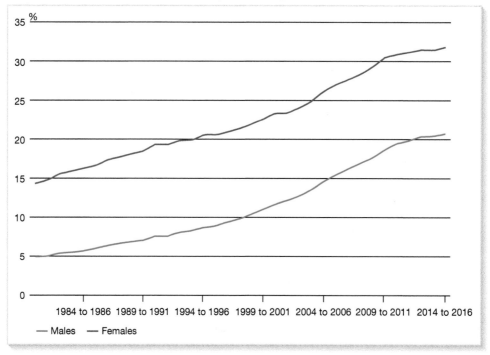

Introduction to epidemiology

Epidemiology is the analysis of patterns, causes and effects of health and disease in defined populations.

By using data on health information, nurses can better understand the incidence, distribution and ways of preventing and managing ill health and disease. Epidemiological information can support nurses' knowledge of how often diseases occur in different groups of people and suggest why this is so. In addition it can support the planning and evaluation strategies to provide support and health care to populations and groups. The analysis of the distribution and determinants of health (described in Unit 1, Chapter 3), in defined populations can answer the question why some groups are more healthy than others.

There are a number of ways in which health information can be gathered. In the UK every 10 years the Office for National Statistics (ONS, 2011), through census gathering, provides a comprehensive insight into the population and the way that it lives.

Demographic information from the census includes statistics on:

- Age
- Gender
- Ethnicity
- Migration
- Mortality
- Birth rates
- Marital status.

The census also taps into self-analysis of individuals' health by asking people to report their general health as either 'very good' or 'good'. Analysis showed a positive outcome in the 2011 census.

Public Health Profiles have been produced annually since 2006 and provide an overview of health for each local authority in England. Nurses can find out about the health profile of any area by using the online interactive maps. The data use health indicators including factors that affect health and disease. These include incidence of violent crime, obesity, deaths from drug misuse, homelessness, infant mortality and lifestyle. To review health profiles by area, go to the Public Health Profiles page on the Public Health England website (http://fingertips.phe.org.uk/).

Epidemiologists study the distribution and causes of health and ill health in populations. The complexity of epidemiology can be demonstrated in Figure 1.6.1. In order to focus on the prevention of ill health and disease, studies focus on four domains:

- Biological determinants, such as age, gender, genetic makeup.
- Environmental determinants, such as housing, green space, access to transport and health care.
- Social determinants, such as income, education, social class.
- Lifestyle determinants, such as health behaviours, exercise, smoking, alcohol consumption, attitudes towards uptake of screening.

Mortality

Bizarrely one of the most accurate means of evaluating health is through the study of death, and mortality data for England and Wales are obtained via the Office for National Statistics (in Scotland via the NHS Scotland Chief Executive's Annual Report, and for Northern Ireland the Annual Report of the Registrar General for Northern Ireland).

Deaths are broken down by age, gender, area and cause of death sourced from the death register. The ONS reports the following from analysis in 2015:

- There were 529 655 deaths registered in England and Wales in 2015, an increase of 5.6% compared with 2014.
- Age-standardised mortality rates (ASMRs) increased in 2015 by 5.1% for females and 3.1% for males – a change to the general decrease in rates in recent years.
- In 2015, mortality rates for respiratory diseases (including flu) increased notably for both males and females.
- Cancer was the most common broad cause of death (28% of all deaths registered) followed by circulatory diseases, such as heart disease and strokes (26%).
- The infant mortality rate remained at 3.9 deaths per 1000 live births in 2015.

To allow comparisons of the number of deaths, the statistics are presented as rates per 1000 of the population in a group and include:

- *The numerator*: number of people who died.
- *The denominator*: the total number of people in the population.
- *The time period*: over what time the deaths took place.

By using death rates epidemiologists can identify modifying factors that can enhance public health and health promotion activities. For example, where evidence points to increased mortality due to influenza in a specified age group, targeted health education and prevention can support a reduction in mortality rates.

The Standardised Mortality Rate (SMR) compares death rates between different populations and is quoted either as a ratio or a percentage. The Age Standardised Mortality Rate (ASMR) for the UK in 2014 was 968.3 deaths per 100 000. In the same time frame, Glasgow had an ASMR of 1380.6. deaths per 100 000 of the population, or 1.4 times the average UK number.

Life expectancy

Measurements of life expectancy use estimates of the population's health and the number of deaths (Figure 1.6.2). Other variables are considered in the estimation of life expectancy; the factors and determinants of health play a huge role. According to the ONS (2016) in 2012 to 2014, life expectancy for newborn baby boys was highest in Kensington and Chelsea (83.3 years) and lowest in Blackpool (74.7 years). For newborn baby girls, life expectancy was highest in Chiltern (86.7 years) and lowest in Middlesbrough (79.8 years).

Public health outcomes and the role of the nurse

Figure 1.7.1 Six key areas in which nurses can impact on personalised care and population health.
Source: Department of Health & Public Health England (2014). Licensed under Open Government Licence v3.0. http://www.nationalarchives.gov.uk/doc/open-government-licence/version/3/.

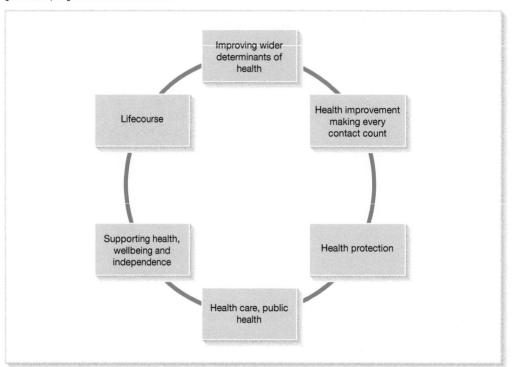

Table 1.7.1 Nursing and Midwifery Council competences that relate directly to aspects of public health work. Source: NMC (2015). http://www.nmc.org.uk/globalassets/sitedocuments/standards/nmc-standards-for-competence-for-registered-nurses.pdf.

Field of nursing	Practice domain	Standard (and page number in document *NMC standards for competence for registered nurses* – NMC, 2015)
Adult	**Communication and interpersonal skills**	Adult nurses must demonstrate the ability to listen with empathy. They must be able to respond warmly and positively to people of all ages who may be anxious, distressed, or facing problems with their health and wellbeing (p. 10)
Children and young people	**Nursing practice and decision making**	'include health promotion, and illness and injury prevention, in their nursing practice. They must promote early intervention to address the links between early life adversity and adult ill health, and the risks to the current and future physical, mental, emotional and sexual health of children and young people' (p. 13)
Learning disability	**Professional values**	'recognise that people with learning disabilities are full and equal citizens, and must promote their health and wellbeing by focusing on and developing their strengths and abilities' (p. 15)
Mental health	**Nursing practice and decision making**	'work to promote mental health, help prevent mental health problems in at-risk groups, and enhance the health and wellbeing of people with mental health problems' (p. 18)

The UK government's Public Health Outcomes Framework (PHOF) for England 2013–2016 has two main aims. It seeks to address the overall population health (increasing the number of years spent free from any physical or mental health disability) and also to address the health inequalities observed between different population groups in England (in terms of life expectancy, incidence and prevalence of different conditions and diseases, numbers of years spent living with a long-term condition or disability, choices available in relation to health). The Framework developed a number of indicators designed to support measurement of progress towards achieving these aims. The indicators are continually reviewed and further developed and can be accessed via the Public Health England (PHE) pages of the GOV.UK website. These indicators relate to four different domains:

- Improving the wider determinants of health
- Health improvement
- Health protection
- Health care, public health and preventing premature mortality.

Chapter 1 of this unit pointed out how two of these domains relate directly to the work that all nurses engage in with every patient/client/service user. This chapter will look at the nurse's role in relation to all these domains and others developed as part of the Framework for Personalised Care and Population Health for Nurses, Midwives, Health Visitors and Allied Health Professionals, released initially in 2014 to identify and support the impact that nurses and others can have in addressing the two main aims of the PHOF referred to above. This framework responds to the changing nature of health and illness in England today, recognising that ill health and disease are more likely to result from the determinants of health referred to in Chapter 3 of this Unit than from the communicable diseases responsible for a very large proportion of the morbidity and mortality rates seen up to the mid-twentieth century. It aims to support and shape what it refers to as 'health promoting practice' at both individual and population level, across the whole life course and in all care environments. It identifies the evidence base that nurses and others can draw on to support their practice. It also recognises that nurses and others can play a large role in influencing and creating a culture for health. Davies et al. (2014) describe this culture as one in which healthy behaviours are the norm and in which 'the institutional, social, and physical environment support this mindset' (p. 1891).

The Nursing and Midwifery Council recognises different aspects of public health to be competencies required of **all** registered nurses (see Box 1.1.1), and Table 1.7.1 of this chapter illustrates this further with reference to specific competencies required by practitioners in the different fields of nursing practice (NMC, 2015).

The Framework for Personalised Care and Population Health looks at six key areas of health promoting practice (Figure 1.7.1).

Wider determinants of health

Nurses can work with patients/clients to mitigate the impact of the determinants of health. This might be through raising someone's awareness of the factors influencing their health and signposting people to ongoing support to manage this influence.

Health improvement: MECC – making every contact count

Along with all workers who have regular contact with the public, nurses are encouraged to give opportunistic, appropriate and timely advice on wellbeing to people they engage with as part of their role. Nurses are ideally placed to do this because of the therapeutic relationships that they develop with people. The Framework encourages the use of National Institute for Health and Care Excellence (NICE) guidance on interventions shown to be successful in supporting individuals to change behaviour in respect of smoking, physical exercise and alcohol use.

Health protection

Programmes aimed at improving both individual and population health, such as immunisation programmes, effective hand washing programmes and contact tracing of people who may be at risk of a communicable disease, are programmes to which nurses can contribute in raising awareness, direct involvement and follow-up.

Health care: public health

The way in which health care services are organised and delivered can impact on the ability of individuals and communities to engage with them. The 'culture' that nurses convey to people needs to be one that conveys health as described above.

Supporting health, wellbeing and independence

Patients generally want to be able to manage their health and manage any illness or long-term condition that they experience. Nurses should always work to create patient independence and should be continually aware of the health of their patients' carers.

Life course

It is important to recognise the different health challenges that people may face at different stages of their lifespan and the different nature of the support that may be needed.

These six activities and examples of them will be referred to in future Units (see Units 3, 4 and 5). Units 3 and 4 will also explore the skills and qualities that nurses should develop to be able to practise in this health-promoting way with all patients. The main skills required are listed below.

Skills/qualities needed by nurses to engage with these six activities

- Self-awareness and emotional intelligence – see Unit 4.
- Knowledge and understanding of the different determinants of health and their impact on individuals and communities – see Unit 3.
- Theoretical knowledge and skill in application of models of behaviour change – Unit 4.
- Access to relevant health profiles – see Unit 3.

8 The prevention of premature mortality: screening

Figure 1.8.1 Screening. Source: UK National Screening Committee. Licensed under Open Government Licence v3.0.http://www.nationalarchives.gov.uk/doc/open-government-licence/version/3/.

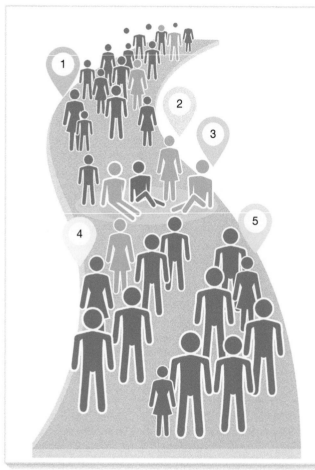

1. These people are offered the screening test

2. These people have decided to have the screening test

3. People caught in the screening sieve have been identified as possibly having the condition being screened for and will therefore be offered further investigations

   (only the people in pink actually have the condition and have been correctly identified the others are unaffected by the condition and are turned fabe positive results)

4. These people have not been picked out as high risk by the screening test so will not go on to further tests or investigations. This does not mean they have no risk but have the same risks as the rest of the population.

   (the person in pink does have the condition being screened for and has slipped through the screening not unidentified – this is bettered a 'fake negative result')

5. Some people may decide not to have the screening test

Table 1.8.1 The criteria for screening.

The disease	Is it an important health problem?
	Is the natural history well understood?
	Is there a long time between the presence of risk factors/subclinical disease to overt disease?
	Does early intervention improve clinical/public health outcome?
Screening test	Is the test valid (sensitivity and specificity)?
	Is the test simple, reliable and affordable?
	Is the test acceptable to patient and staff?
Diagnosis and treatment	Is access to diagnostic facilities available and rapid?
	Is treatment effective and accessible?
	Is it cost-effective?
	Is it sustainable?
	Does benefit outweigh the harm?

Introduction

Screening is a method adopted within public health to identify individuals who are outwardly healthy, but who may be at risk of disease or ill health. In this way members of a defined group or population can be identified by means of testing to realistically assess the risk of or find undiagnosed health problems. The process of screening is not 100% perfect, and in every screening programme there will be a number of false positives and false negatives.

Screening can offer suitable preventative intervention, either **primary** or **secondary**:

• Primary prevention is aimed at preventing the development of disease, e.g. body mass index (BMI) assessment.
• Secondary prevention is aimed at preventing the serious outcome of existing disease, e.g. breast cancer screening.

Examples of screening for health-related conditions in the UK are varied and can be directly related to particular aspects of health, such as an individual's age, gender, ethnic background, their occupation and so on. Figure 1.8.2 [see appendix] demonstrates a timeline for common health screening activities within the UK. Here you can identify target groups according to age where screening can only be effective if targeted at a certain time in a person's life.

Examples of age appropriate screening are:

• The Newborn Blood Spot (NBS) screening programme, which aims to identify rare conditions at birth that can lead to serious illness, developmental delay or even infant mortality. Further information can be sourced on the NHS Choices website (nhs.uk/bloodspot).
• The NHS Bowel Cancer Screening Programme (BCSP) aims to target individuals every two years who are between the ages of 60 to 74 with the offer of an occult blood sampling kit. Other screening activities include bowel scope screening to all men and women in England aged 55.

Examples of gender appropriate screening are:

• The Cervical Screening Programme (CSP), which is available to women over the age of 25. This aims to identify evidence of cervical cancer and the presence of the human papilloma virus (HPV).
• The Abdominal Aortic Aneurysm (AAA) screening test is offered to men in their 65th year.

An example of occupational screening is:

• Hepatitis B screening for health care workers.

Screening can fall into a number of categories.

• **Selective** screening is applied to specific target groups who may be identified because of behaviour or risk, e.g. screening people with diabetes for evidence of diabetic retinopathy.
• **Mass** screening invites all regardless of risk for systematic testing. Examples include mammography, where the aim is to test large numbers of people without regard to their individual risk factors.
• Screening can be **routine**, e.g. prenatal and postnatal testing, or can be **genetic**, when used to identify risk of inherited or existing conditions.
• **Anonymous** screening can be used without permission to establish disease patterns within a given population group.
• **Opportunistic** screening can occur at the interface between the nurse and the individual and can involve very simple non-invasive assessments of, e.g. BMI, or more advanced screening such as blood lipid analysis or lung function screening.

The screening sieve

Figures 1.8.1 represents the screening sieve. Here you can see that most people pass through the sieve, demonstrating a low risk of the disease or condition being screened for. Those left in the sieve have a higher risk, and further investigation, diagnostic testing or treatment is offered to them.

At every stage of the test, individuals can choose future options of tests, treatments, advice and support.

Criteria for screening

Screening activities should be open to evaluation in relation to their effectiveness, viability and appropriateness.

• The disease or health-related condition should be identifiable by the screening test.
• Early identification and/or treatment should be able to improve the outcome for individuals or groups.
• The test should be **specific** (this relates to the proportion of people free from disease who are tested: a test that is highly specific will give a high level of false negatives); and be evaluated as to its **sensitivity** (this relates to the degree of false positive results: a highly sensitive test will result in a high number of false positive results).
• It should be cost effective.

Table 1.8.1 identifies and demonstrates the criteria for screening.

Nurses need to be aware of the need for careful support to help individuals who are outwardly healthy to make informed choices about agreeing to screening, and to support individuals through the screening process. Individuals need opportunities to explore their expectations of what screening can offer them;

Screening can significantly improve the quality of an individual's life through early risk analysis and reduce the risk of major ill health. However, screening cannot guarantee protection in the future, it can only analyse risk and/or the presence of disease.

9 Health surveillance

Figure 1.9.1 The wider determinants of health. Source: Dahlgren and Whitehead (1991).

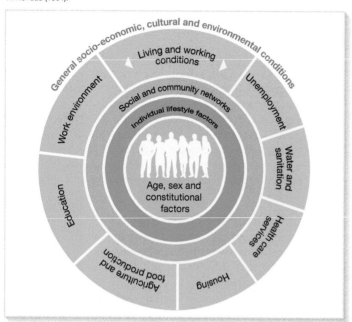

Box 1.9.1 Case study.

Marianna, a 57-year-old Nigerian woman, is invited to the GP surgery for a general health check-up. The following information will be recorded:

- Her weight
- Waist measurement
- Blood pressure and pulse
- Smoking status
- Alcohol consumption, drug use now and in the past
- Her family medical history
- Her dietary habits
- Her physical activity
- Blood analysis for cholesterol levels, haemoglobiin A1C (HbA1C) test, full blood count (FBC) and electrolyte tests
- Her postcode, which can be an indication of her socioeconomic status
- Ethnicity
- Employment status, which can indicate social class
- Marital/partnership status

Table 1.9.1 Causative agents notifiable to Public Health England under the Health Protection (Notification) Regulations (2010). Source: Public Health England. Licensed under Open Government Licence v3.0. http://www.nationalarchives.gov.uk/doc/open-government-licence/version/3/.

Bacillus anthracis	Entamoeba histolytica	Omsk haemorrhagic fever virus
Bacillus cereus (only if associated with food poisoning)	Francisella tularensis	Plasmodium falciparum, vivax, ovale, malariae, knowlesi
Bordetella pertussis	Giardia lamblia	Polio virus (wild or vaccine types)
Borrelia spp.	Guanarito virus	Rabies virus (classical rabies and rabies-related lyssaviruses)
Brucella spp.	Haemophilus influenzae (invasive)	Rickettsia spp.
Burkholderia mallei	Hanta virus	Rift Valley fever virus
Burkholderia pseudomallei	Hepatitis A, B, C, delta, and E viruses	Rubella virus
Campylobacter spp.	Influenza virus	Sabia virus
Chikungunya virus	Junin virus	Salmonella spp.
Chlamydophila psittaci	Kyasanur Forest disease virus	SARS coronavirus
Clostridium botulinum	Lassa virus	Shigella spp.
Clostridium perfringens (only if associated with food poisoning)	Legionella spp.	Streptococcus pneumoniae (invasive)
Clostridium tetani	Leptospira interrogans	Streptococcus pyogenes (invasive)
Corynebacterium diphtheriae	Listeria monocytogenes	Varicella zoster virus
Corynebacterium ulcerans	Machupo virus	Variola virus
Coxiella burnetii	Marburg virus	Verocytotoxigenic Escherichia coli (including E. coli O157)
Crimean-Congo haemorrhagic fever virus	Measles virus	Vibrio cholerae
Cryptosporidium spp.	Mumps virus	West Nile Virus
Dengue virus	Mycobacterium tuberculosis complex	Yellow fever virus
Ebola virus	Neisseria meningitidis	Yersinia pestis

Public Health and Health Promotion for Nurses at a Glance, First Edition. Karen Wild and Maureen McGrath.
© 2019 John Wiley & Sons Ltd. Published 2019 by John Wiley & Sons Ltd.

According to the World Health Organization, public health surveillance is: 'the continuous, systematic collection, analysis and interpretation of health-related data needed for the planning, implementation, and evaluation of public health practice. Such surveillance can:

• serve as an early warning system for impending public health emergencies;

• document the impact of requirements an intervention, or track progress towards specified goals; and

• monitor and clarify the epidemiology of health problems, to allow priorities to be set and to inform public health policy and strategies' (World Health Organization, 2016).

Surveillance of health

Statistics around health and ill health are collected and reported in a variety of ways. Acute and longer term health trends can be measured; these take into account the many determinants of health. Acute illness trends, such as communicable diseases, tend to focus on the physiological aspects of illness; for example, all laboratories in England performing a primary diagnostic role must notify Public Health England when they confirm a notifiable organism. Table 1.9.1 shows the current list of notifiable diseases. Medical practitioners registered within England and Wales have a statutory duty to notify their local authority or local Health Protection Team of suspected cases of certain infectious diseases.

Long-term conditions affecting health and wellbeing focus on the wider determinants of health and are drawn from examples of data highlighted in Figure 1.9.1. These can be gathered throughout the lifespan, and rely on careful and accurate data collection. Standard mortality ratios (SMRs) can be used to analyse death by cause. Early deaths (below average life expectancy) are considered premature and therefore to a degree preventable. These data are collected en masse and also at an individual level as part of collective screening programmes.

In the case study in Box 1.9.1, Marianna is assessed to check her risk of heart disease, diabetes, stroke and kidney disease. The risk assessment will result in a risk score, and provides an ideal opportunity for the nurse to engage in supporting Marianna in improving her health and referring her to local support services.

Health outcomes

Patients have a right to know about the outcome of health surveillance, and an open dialogue can support better awareness and understanding from both the individual's perspective and that of the nurse. In the case study, Marianna may gain an insight into her 'heart age', and modifiable and non-modifiable risk factors can be highlighted and focused on to inform her future health.

Population or group health surveillance can better inform local health care provision. Annual public health reports are available that highlight local trends in health, the SMR rates and the social determinants of health in an area. Go to Health Profiles on the GOV.UK website (www.gov.uk/government/collections/health-profiles) to download the results of health surveillance in your geographical area. Such health profiles give the reader summary health information, which can be used as an effective tool for health improvement.

Using health information

An understanding of the epidemiological information and risk factors associated with acute and long-term health problems helps the nurse to engage in health promotional activities. Awareness of the wider determinants of health that contribute to health outcomes is essential. Understanding the varied resources that are available to survey and report on health helps the nurse to prioritise health care needs of communities and to identify broader public health requirements, and appropriate intervention. In the case study (Box 1.9.1), it may be appropriate to offer Marianne a 'prescription' for exercise and weight loss, with free access to a local gym and reduced fees at a slimming club. Skills in applying evidence-based health promotion, seeking and analysing data, and applying findings within the clinical setting underpin the nurse's role in using health information (Wills, 2014).

10 Inequalities in health

Figure 1.10.1 Inequalities in health.

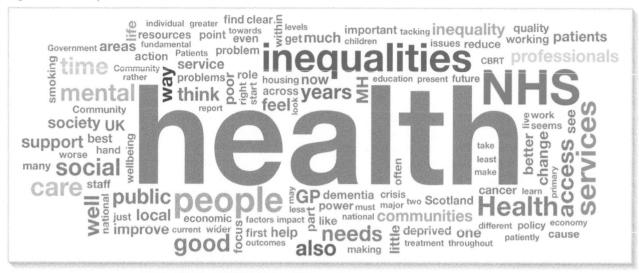

Figure 1.10.2 Smoking and deprivation. Source: Public Health England. https://www.gov.uk/government/publications/health-matters-smoking-and-quitting-in-england/smoking-and-quitting-in-england. Licensed under Open Comment [RH1]: Government Licence v3.0. http://www.nationalarchives.gov.uk/doc/open-government-licence/version/3/.

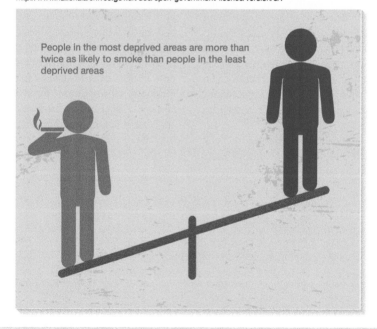

People in the most deprived areas are more than twice as likely to smoke than people in the least deprived areas

Public Health and Health Promotion for Nurses at a Glance, First Edition. Karen Wild and Maureen McGrath.
© 2019 John Wiley & Sons Ltd. Published 2019 by John Wiley & Sons Ltd.

Inequality and social class

Current opinions about the underlying causes of health inequalities are divided, but their common aim is to explain the reasons why groups in society might be affected. In Figure 1.10.1 you can see the arguments put forward to demonstrate two ideas around the causes of inequality: the psychosocial and neo-material perspectives.

A third explanation is offered by the **life course** account of inequality (this is explored more fully in Unit 1, Chapter 11); it provides an alternative viewpoint as to why there are such differences in health, and supports the notion that health effects of adverse socioeconomic circumstances accumulate throughout the life course. The proposition is that the effects of poverty are strongest in those who are born, grow up in, and remain in material hardship, and this is manifest in the next generation – the so-called 'cycle of poverty'.

People in the UK have traditionally been classified socially as being upper, middle or lower class, and defined by occupation, wealth and education. The Registrar General's social classification was based on occupation and ranged from professional occupations, such as doctors, to unskilled occupations, such as labourers.

These stereotypes of the twentieth century are seen as outdated, and sociologists are inclined to view class in relation to cultural and social activities, as well as wealth. Research from the BBC Lab UK (BBC News, 2013) suggests that class has three dimensions:

- Economic capital – which considers such aspects as a person's income, savings and house value.
- Social capital – which looks at the number and status of people that a person knows socially.
- Cultural capital – defined as the extent and nature of cultural interests and activities that a person engages in.

What emerges is the suggestion of a revision of the established way of classifying people socially, as shown in Figure 1.10.2.

Compare Figure 1.10.2 with the Office for National Statistics (ONS) classification, which has its categories aggregated to produce approximate social classes I–V, as follows:

I Professional occupations
II Managerial and technical occupations
III Skilled occupations
IV Partly skilled occupations
V Unskilled occupations.

Whatever method of classification is used to determine social class, one constant remains: those who are socioeconomically less well off tend to have poorer health, and this can be because of their living or working conditions, resources and their social effect, lifestyle issues or any combination of these factors.

Public Health England has an interactive map that highlights premature mortality across every local authority area (http://healthierlives.phe.org.uk/topic/mortality). This demonstrates the best and worst geographical locations for risk of premature death in the UK. Click on the map to see the ranking out of 150 for your area. The highest scores relate to the worst areas for risk of premature death.

Poverty is a central concern of public health, not only in this country but also worldwide. People living in poverty (this can equate to poor housing, overcrowding, and poor sanitary conditions) have a reduced life expectancy and experience poorer health than the rest of the population.

The housing conditions that are proven to be important for health include:

- Overcrowding (linked to infectious/respiratory disease).
- Damp and mould (linked to respiratory disease, eczema, asthma and rhinitis), indoor pollutants and infestation (linked to asthma).
- Low temperature (linked to respiratory infection, hypothermia, bronchospasm and heart disease).
- Homelessness (linked to a range of conditions).
- Unpopular, stigmatised or poor housing and neighbourhood conditions (linked to poor mental health) (Marsh et al., 2010)

While poverty is synonymous with health breakdown, it does not always follow that pattern. The evidence on drug use and alcohol consumption suggests that both are widespread in society; for the most part, consumption bears little relationship to social class or income. Marmot (1997) presents evidence for 'heavy' drinking (those regularly drinking above the recommended daily allowance) that shows lower levels of heavy consumption among unemployed people than among those in work, with the greatest incidence among those in professional and managerial occupations. He concludes that survey evidence does not 'lend support to the popular conception that it is the poor and unemployed who are disproportionately represented among heavy drinkers'.

Similarly, data on drug use show that, while experimentation with drugs is widespread among young people (half of all 16–24-year-olds report having used drugs at some time), there is little variation by socioeconomic circumstances or correlation with poverty and social exclusion.

Investigations into inequalities in health: reports and reviews

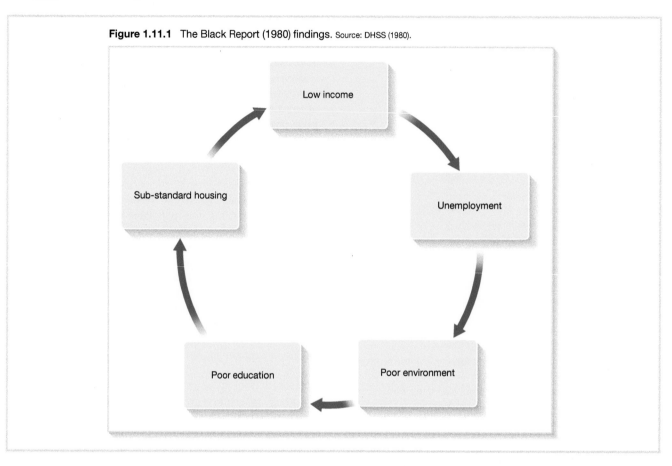

Figure 1.11.1 The Black Report (1980) findings. Source: DHSS (1980).

Low income

Unemployment

Poor environment

Poor education

Sub-standard housing

Public Health and Health Promotion for Nurses at a Glance, First Edition. Karen Wild and Maureen McGrath.
© 2019 John Wiley & Sons Ltd. Published 2019 by John Wiley & Sons Ltd.

The Black Report

In 1998, the government commissioned a report into health inequalities, which was carried out by Sir Donald Acheson. The report emphasised the importance of the social and economic environment as a factor in health inequalities (Acheson, 1998). Figure 1.11.1 highlights the main inequalities that the report identified.

There are a number of organisations that support research and development to investigate the causes of health inequalities. While many are government-led and supported, some are independent charitable organisations.

The Joseph Rowntree Foundation and Housing Trust is a dual charity that aims to:
• **Search** out the underlying causes of poverty and inequality, and identify solutions – through research and learning from experience.
• **Demonstrate** solutions – by developing and running services, stewardship of our land and buildings, innovating and supporting others to innovate.
• **Influence** positive and lasting change – publishing and promoting evidence, and bringing people together to share ideas.

In order to deliver appropriate health services to local communities, it is important that the make-up and needs of the population are understood. It is widely recognised that health status is dependent upon the 'wider determinants of health', which are measured using indicators of deprivation.

The Marmot Review

In November 2008, Professor Sir Michael Marmot was asked by the Secretary of State for Health to chair an independent review to set objectives for the most effective evidence-based strategies for reducing health inequalities in England from 2010.

Published on 11 February 2010, it proposed an evidence-based strategy to address the social determinants of health, the conditions in which people are born, grow up, live, work and age, and that can lead to health inequalities. It draws further attention to the evidence that most people in England are not living as long as the most well off in society and spend longer in ill health.

The detailed report contains many important findings, some of which are summarised below:
• People living in the poorest neighbourhoods in England will on average die seven years earlier than people living in the richest neighbourhoods.
• People living in poorer areas not only die sooner, but spend more of their lives with disability – an average total difference of 17 years.

The Review highlights the social gradient of health inequalities – put simply, the lower one's social and economic status, the poorer one's health is likely to be. Health inequalities arise from a complex interaction of many factors – housing, income, education, social isolation, disability – all of which can be strongly affected by one's economic and social status.

Health inequalities are largely preventable. Not only is there a strong social justice case for addressing health inequalities, but also there is a pressing economic case. It is estimated that the annual cost of health inequalities is between £36 billion and £40 billion through lost taxes, welfare payments and costs to the NHS. Action on health inequalities requires action across all the social determinants of health, including education, occupation, income, home and community.

The objectives propose six interventions that address the social determinants of health inequalities (Marmot, 2010):
1 Give every child the best start in life.
2 Enable all children, young people and adults to maximise their capabilities and have control over their lives.
3 Create fair employment and good work for all.
4 Ensure a healthy standard of living for all.
5 Create and develop healthy and sustainable places and communities.
6 Strengthen the role and impact of ill health prevention.

Future challenges for the NHS concern the demand for health care and provision and the supply of health and social services. The demand for health care is increasing because of an ageing society, a rise in the incidence of long-term conditions, and an increase in the expectations of the public. The supply of health care is challenged because of increasing costs of providing care combined with constraints on public resources.

12 The relationship between public health and competency standards for registered nurses

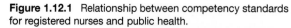

Figure 1.12.1 Relationship between competency standards for registered nurses and public health.

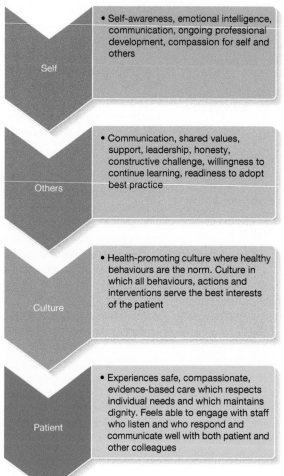

Self
- Self-awareness, emotional intelligence, communication, ongoing professional development, compassion for self and others

Others
- Communication, shared values, support, leadership, honesty, constructive challenge, willingness to continue learning, readiness to adopt best practice

Culture
- Health-promoting culture where healthy behaviours are the norm. Culture in which all behaviours, actions and interventions serve the best interests of the patient

Patient
- Experiences safe, compassionate, evidence-based care which respects individual needs and which maintains dignity. Feels able to engage with staff who listen and who respond and communicate well with both patient and other colleagues

Public Health and Health Promotion for Nurses at a Glance, First Edition. Karen Wild and Maureen McGrath.
© 2019 John Wiley & Sons Ltd. Published 2019 by John Wiley & Sons Ltd.

Competency standards for registered nurses

In 2014 the Nursing and Midwifery Council (NMC) published a document that outlined the standards of clinical competence that all nurses must meet on qualification and that they must maintain throughout their careers (NMC, 2014). This document aligns closely with the Standards for Pre-registration Nursing Education (NMC, 2010). This latter document is due to be updated and made available by late 2018. This review of undergraduate education standards is unlikely to dramatically change the standards of competence required of all qualified nurses referred to here and reflected in NHS England's new framework for nursing, midwifery and care staff (NHS England, 2016) and in the Francis Report (The Mid-Staffordshire NHS Foundation Trust Public Inquiry, 2013).

The document outlines generic competencies that apply across all fields of nursing, and specific competencies relating to the separate fields of Adult Nursing, Mental Health Nursing, Learning Disabilities Nursing and Children's Nursing. For the purpose of this chapter we will look at how the concepts of public health and health promotion relate to the generic competencies. The competencies are considered under four main areas of professional practice

- Professional values
- Communication and interpersonal skills
- Nursing practice and decision making
- Leadership, management and teamworking.

Professional values

Under this area of practice nurses are expected to demonstrate accountability for safe, compassionate, person-centred care that is based on sound evidence and that respects the dignity and human rights of all others. They are expected to work in partnership with patients and other professionals to ensure all decision making is shared.

If a nurse is working to promote health with an individual patient a relationship of trust and mutual respect needs to be developed. This relationship will necessarily be patient or client centred, and the nurse will aim to understand the context within which health is being promoted, whether this be supporting someone to manage a complex medication regime, reduce alcohol intake, learn a basic personal care skill or attend an immunisation appointment. An approach that encourages individual agency rather than one that informs and directs is respectful of the dignity and human rights of patients and clients.

Communication and interpersonal skills

These skills are seen as central to all nursing competence. Nurses are expected to communicate safely, effectively, compassionately and respectfully with **everyone** whom they come into contact with professionally. The use of a range of communication strategies is seen as essential. Nurses must be able to recognise the need for, and to also implement reasonable adjustments in order to provide optimum care for anyone with any kind of disability.

Excellent communication skills underpin all health promotion and public health work. In order to engage individuals or communities in any aspect of public health, whether this is related to the wider determinants of health (in terms of developing resilience against their impact or challenging their impact politically), improving health, engaging in programmes and practices to protect health or developing services to promote a culture of health, nurses have to listen in order to really understand health from the perspective of the person/community they are working with, and not from the perspective of service or government policy. Unit 4 in this book will look in detail at the complex communication skills nurses may use to support health improvement and health gain.

Nursing practice and decision making

All nurses are expected to be able to competently assess and meet the full range of essential physical and mental health needs of people of all ages. They should be able to provide safe and effective immediate care where necessary and should be able to understand and address complex and coexisting needs. The impact of behaviour, culture, socioeconomic and other factors on health and on recovery from illness must be taken account of.

Chapter 3 of this Unit has explored the impact of the wider determinants of health that must always be taken account of in any health promotion activity at individual or community level, and this will be explored further in Units 2 and 4.

Leadership, management and team working

Under this area of practice nurses are expected to respond appropriately to planned and uncertain situations, managing themselves and others effectively. They are expected to evaluate care and shape future practice as a result. Nurses should identify priorities and manage time and resources effectively. The importance of self-awareness and recognition of the impact that their own values, principles and assumptions may have on practice and on others is indicated. The coordination, delegation and supervision of care is stressed as a key competency.

Nurses who are working with people to promote health need to recognise when people are ready to engage with this kind of care and support. They need skills to be able to assess a person's readiness to change and be able to discuss this with them. Delegation or referral to other services may be appropriate until the person feels ready to look at making changes.

The competency standards for nurses are clearly reflected in the best of public health and health-promoting practice. It is key that healthy behaviours are reflected in individual nurses and within nursing teams in order to create a culture of health in which the needs of the patient come first in every decision made about care (Figure 1.12.1).

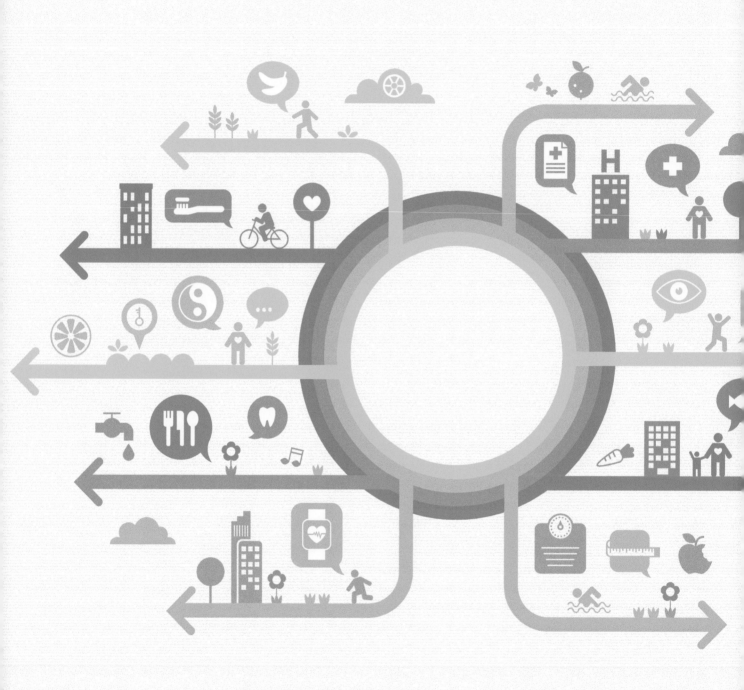

What has health promotion to do with nursing?

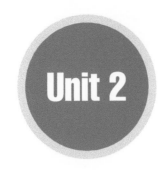

Unit 2

Chapters

Thinking points for NMC Revalidation

In Unit 2 you will have learnt what health promotion is and how nurses engage in health promotion activities. Think of recent encounters with your patient group, and consider how you might distinguish between health education and health promotion activities.

1 Health promotion

Table 2.1.1 Three key pillars of health promotion. Source: World Health Organization (2016).

Three pillars of health promotion	What this means
Pillar 1 Good governance	Health is determined by multiple factors outside the direct control of the health sector
	Laws, statutes and policies should all be designed and implemented in ways that make healthy choices easier for all members of society irrespective of social, economic or health status. Public and private organisations should develop sustainable structures and services that enable contribution from and collaboration with all members of society
Pillar 2 Healthy cities	Globally more people live in urban areas than in rural settings
	Cities should be managed and planned in ways that advance health and health equity. Thought must be given to developing environmental, physical and social environments which support health and the maximisation of individual and community potential
Pillar 3 Health literacy	Health literacy is an important resource in addressing inequities in health
	Individuals and communities should have access to knowledge and skills to enable them to make healthy decisions and choices. There needs to be creative development of different ways of accessing and using knowledge that will take account of the variety of needs in different individuals and communities

Public Health and Health Promotion for Nurses at a Glance, First Edition. Karen Wild and Maureen McGrath.
© 2019 John Wiley & Sons Ltd. Published 2019 by John Wiley & Sons Ltd.

An emphasis on promoting good health in contrast to treating illness or health breakdown was first proposed in the 1970s. This was due to recognition of the rising costs of health care as life expectancies started to increase and health technologies and pharmacology developed further. In addition there was a recognised shift in the major causes of mortality and morbidity away from infectious diseases to chronic diseases associated with health behaviours. This period was also one in which a number of movements, such as feminism, community development and self help, were challenging societal structures that embraced the dominance of class and gender-related power.

Within medicine and health there was a challenge for patients to own their own health and to be treated as partners in their health care, able to make decisions about health and illness. This led initially to a burgeoning of information about health and the body made available to people through mass communication methods as well as booklets and leaflets designed to be used by patients with particular health needs. This was called 'health education' and was aimed at informing people about the impact of some health behaviours on the body. This idea was a good one in that none of us are able to make a decision about our health or about how best to manage a chronic illness unless we have knowledge that relates to it. However, it was recognised that information alone is not always enough to prevent ill health or to maintain and improve health. Unless people are **able** to act on the knowledge they have about factors that impact on health they may feel even more disempowered with knowledge than they were without it. In 1986 the World Health Organization (1986) held the first international conference on health promotion in Ottawa and defined it as:

> the process of enabling people to increase control over and improve their health. Health is seen as a resource for everyday life, not the object of living. Health is not just the responsibility of the health sector but goes beyond healthy lifestyles to wellbeing

This definition encompassed a welcome change of emphasis from an expectation that 'telling' people what to do and how to be would automatically improve health, to the idea that everything in a person's life and environment impacts on their health and on the control they have over health experience. It also suggests that people might enjoy health – in the sense of wellbeing – even in the presence of ill health or disability. For nurses working with people to promote health this definition underpins a way of working that places an emphasis on what the patient wants (in the sense of developing resources for living) and what will best help them to positively experience different aspects of their individual, family and social life.

The World Health Organization has held international/global conferences on health promotion in subsequent years – the most recent being the 2016 conference held in Shanghai. This conference strongly linked health promotion with sustainable development, and identified three key elements of health promotion: good governance; health literacy (in the sense of people having the knowledge, skills and information to make healthy choices **as well as** the opportunity to act on those choices); and healthy cities. Table 2.1.1 summarises these elements. The conference explored a range of 17 topics such as prioritising the health needs of the poor, supporting low-carbon developments, sustaining fish stocks and promoting wellbeing for all ages. The issue here is that health promotion appears to relate to anything and everything and this can make it feel less relevant to the day-to-day work of many nurses. This may be why many nurses feel comfortable with health education as opposed to health promotion. The giving of a leaflet is a tangible and arguably relevant way of 'helping' someone without impacting greatly on the valuable resource of time.

Resources to support health promotion

As indicated in Unit 1 nurses need to place advice and support given to patients in the context of the individual, family and community environment that they are living in. This **does** take time, and in Unit 4 there is a discussion of techniques that enable nurses to engage with patients in ways that support meaningful health promotion in a relatively short time.

There are a number of useful resources to support nurses working with a range of different patients in order to promote health. In Unit 1 Chapter 7, the Framework for Personalised Care and Population Health (Department of Health and Public Health England, 2014) was considered. This Framework will continue to develop and respond to the changing nature of health and illness in England and the digital first successor is now available. This resource, All Our Health (Public Health England, 2016), aims to shape and support the contribution health professionals make to health promotion by supporting practice and culture that always:
- Prevents avoidable illness
- Protects health
- Promotes wellbeing and resilience.

This is also a response to the new Framework for Nursing and Midwifery – Leading Change, Adding Value (NHS England, 2016), which sets out three (out of a total of ten) commitments to prevention of illness and improving population health. Nurses cannot ignore health promotion whatever their area of practice. Please take some time to access the resources and infographics designed to support nurses and other health-care professionals available on the government website; see the pages under All Our Health (https://www.gov.uk/government/collections/all-our-health-personalised-care-and-population-health).

In the next two chapters we will look at some different aspects of health promotion.

2 Aspects of health promotion

Figure 2.2.1 Tannahill model of health promotion.
Source: Tannahill (2009).

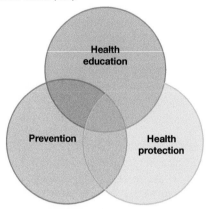

Health education

Prevention

Health protection

Box 2.2.1 Personal and professional attributes of Health Visitors.
Source: GOV.UK (2012, updated 2015) Health Visiting Attributes (p. 2).

- Proactively interested in public health prevention and early intervention.
- Adaptable and influential.
- Respectful of different values, taking a holistic approach to care.
- Insightful when communicating.
- Able to engage others and build partnerships.
- Able to demonstrate professionalism.
- Supportive with an adaptive communication style.

Figure 2.2.2 Beattie model of health promotion. Source: McIlfatrick *et al.*, (2013); adapted from Thomas and Stewart (2004). Reproduced with permission of Sonja McIlfatrick.

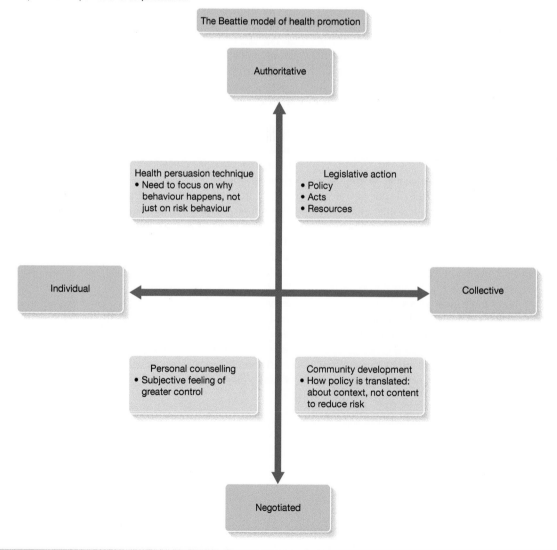

The Beattie model of health promotion

Authoritative

Health persuasion technique
- Need to focus on why behaviour happens, not just on risk behaviour

Legislative action
- Policy
- Acts
- Resources

Individual

Collective

Personal counselling
- Subjective feeling of greater control

Community development
- How policy is translated: about context, not content to reduce risk

Negotiated

Public Health and Health Promotion for Nurses at a Glance, First Edition. Karen Wild and Maureen McGrath.
© 2019 John Wiley & Sons Ltd. Published 2019 by John Wiley & Sons Ltd.

There are a number of different models of health promotion that attempt to incorporate different elements of health promotion practice. Figures 2.2.1 and 2.2.2 and Box 2.2.1 illustrate just three of these. Beattie's (1991) model (Figure 2.2.2) looks at different options for conceptualising and planning health promotion that relates to work either with individuals or communities. The other aspect that this model considers is whether the philosophical approach taken to health promotion should be an authoritative one or a negotiated one. Different issues will require different approaches and will take account of the evidence base on what is effective, the degree of risk posed by a public health issue, and the acceptability and justification of the level of intrusiveness of an approach (Nuffield Council on Bioethics, 2007).

The legislative ban on smoking in public places, which was introduced in England in July 2007, was based on clear evidence regarding the impact of smoking and passive smoking on health and on the fact that the ban was straightforward to effect and monitor. Many smokers were supportive of the ban. It would be very difficult and unacceptable to pass legislation about what people should eat in terms of the portions of fruit and vegetables consumed daily. The evidence on the amounts of fruit and vegetables that make a difference to health is much more complex and is less conclusive. There is a clear association between diet and obesity/cardiovascular disease/cancers but the impact of factors such as food type and eating patterns is very complex and influenced by several (often interacting) variables. Such legislation would also be seen as very intrusive into individual and family lives and would be almost impossible to monitor. However it **is** seen as appropriate to give people advice to eat a healthy diet that regularly incorporates fruit and vegetables.

Box 2.2.1 shows the key personal and professional attributes of Health Visitors who are health promotion practitioners at both individual and community levels. Underpinning all of these attributes is the ability to use a variety of different communication techniques in order to support people in developing practical and realistic ways of improving and maintaining health. These communication techniques will be explored further in Unit 4.

Tannahill's model of health promotion is shown in Figure 2.2.1. This model was developed in 1985 to try to conceptualise the then new construct of health, which then, as now, was a term that seemed to cover so many different ideas as to be meaningless. The model has been criticised as being both simplistic and restricting the idea of health promotion to a medical context of preventing disease. However, the model has currency to this day and has been defended by Tannahill 20 years on from its original development (Tannahill, 2009). It is included here as it is a useful resource for nurses in all fields to understand the need for the different aspects of health promotion that it considers.

Health protection

This is an aspect of health promotion that relates to improving the health of individuals and populations through legal or fiscal measures. The law preventing smoking in public places, which was referred to earlier, is one example of a legal measure aimed at improving health. Others are the legal requirement on medical practitioners to notify local Health Protection Teams of suspected cases of certain notifiable diseases, for example meningitis, poliomyelitis, typhoid and paratyphoid fever, measles and food poisoning. The legal age restriction on the purchase of alcohol to those over 18 years is another example of health protection through legal measures. Fiscal measures are those relating to attempts to improve health through increasing the costs of a practice seen as hazardous to health (e.g. smoking or drinking alcohol) or decreasing the costs of practices seen as improving health such as free or cheaper costs of fitness/swimming classes or free entrance to museums and art galleries. Health protection also relates to those programmes that are organised to offer a service to populations (or to sections of populations) that will protect them from contracting disease or that will help to identify a condition at an early stage. Examples include childhood immunisation programmes, 'flu' vaccinations for adults, and screening programmes such as breast/cervical/vascular/bowel screening. Many would argue that fair welfare benefits and progressive taxation are important aspects of health protection in populations also.

Prevention of ill health

Prevention of ill health can be considered to take place at a number of different levels. Primary prevention is anything aimed at preventing the development of ill health or the symptoms of ill health. Secondary prevention is anything that addresses symptoms of ill health to prevent the development of an established disease or condition. It includes those activities that are aimed at detection of a disease or condition at an early stage. Tertiary prevention is anything aimed at supporting people to live well within the constraints of an established/irreversible condition or disease. These different levels will be explored more in the next chapter.

Health education

Health education at the simplest level is provision of information and knowledge about health and how best to maintain it. Examples are leaflets about healthy diet or safe drinking, pictures of smoking-related disease on cigarette packets, and videos on dental hygiene or memory loss played on a loop while awaiting a GP appointment. Tones and Tilford (1994) described health education as an activity designed to influence values, beliefs and attitudes that may facilitate the acquisition of skills to maintain or improve health. Green and Tones (2010) consider health education to have a central role in contributing to healthy public policy and believe health promotion to be the synergistic relationship between health education and healthy public policy.

Primary and secondary prevention of ill health and health education
1. Cardiovascular disease in men

Figure 2.3.1 Risk factors for high blood pressure. Source: Public Health England. Licensed under Open Government Licence v3.0. http://www. nationalarchives.gov.uk/doc/open-government-licence/version/3/.

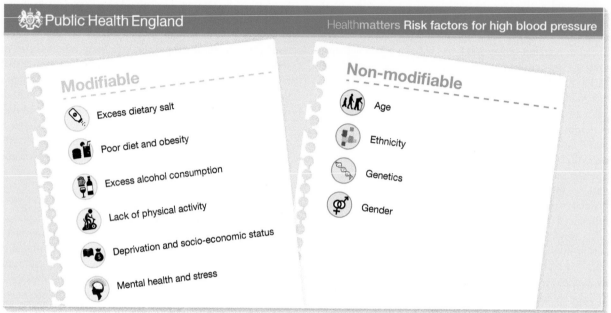

Box 2.3.1 Risk factors for cardiovascular disease.
Source: National Institute for Health and Care Excellence (2016).

- Smoking
- High cholesterol ratio
- Raised blood pressure
- Diabetes
- Inactivity
- Overweight or obesity
- Unhealthy diet
- Depression or isolation

Cardiovascular disease in men

The most recent mortality statistics relating to men of all ages in England and Wales indicate that cardiovascular diseases (CVD), incorporating heart disease and cerebrovascular disease (stroke, transient ischaemia, vascular dementia and subarachnoid haemorrhage), accounted for the majority of registered deaths in 2013 (Office for National Statistics, 2017).

In terms of health protection the NHS Health Check is offered, usually via GP surgeries, to all people aged 40–74. This is an opportunity to be assessed for risk factors such as high blood pressure (BP), body mass index (BMI) and cholesterol ratio – ratio of total cholesterol to high density lipoprotein (HDL) cholesterol – all of which are indicators for risk of cardiovascular disease (Box 2.3.1 and Figure 2.3.1). The ban on smoking in public places aimed at reducing the development of risk factors for CVD is also an example of health protection. Other health protection matters being considered by some local authorities are improving transport options to encourage walking to and from transport points, and limiting the numbers of fast food outlets in areas. Both of these measures are aimed at reducing the obesogenic environment. In addition the Food Standards Agency has been working with food manufacturers to reduce the amounts of salt and sugar added to processed foods.

Primary prevention of cardiovascular diseases in men

Primary prevention of these diseases is about trying to prevent the key risk factors for these diseases – smoking, high blood pressure, high cholesterol ratio and unhealthy weight gain – from developing. The most effective way of doing this is by supporting parents of children to encourage the provision of healthy diets, exercise, smoke-free environments and examples of safe, sensible and social drinking of alcohol. The environment in which children are raised has a key influence on later health behaviours.

Midwives, health visitors and nurses from the Family Nurse Partnership (FNP) programme are ideally placed to help families both in terms of health education and through practical, realistic support and signposting to other agencies that can help them provide a healthy environment in which to raise their family.

Healthy schools and workplaces are also key in preventing the development of the CVD risk factors. Healthy school meals/ snacks, availability of drinking water, provision of supervised regular exercise that children enjoy (e.g. dancing, rollerblading and skateboarding as well as football, netball and athletics) and support on techniques to deal with stress, bullying (both direct and cyberbullying), safeguarding and relationships would all be helpful in reducing the impact of determinants that influence the relevant risk factors in the school environment. Similar provision in workplaces in relation to healthy foods plus information on, and support with, mental health and wellbeing might help maintain health. School nurses and occupational health nurses can be influential in creating healthy school and work environments and in providing support to individuals.

In older people some of the physiological changes associated with ageing will increase the risk of cardiovascular disease, and to date we have no way of preventing this. The vasculature of older people manifests a level of atherosclerosis that has built up over time as the physiological processes that maintain the health of blood vessels become less efficient. This will lead to arterial thickening and stiffness along with endothelial dysfunction and will increase the risk of high blood pressure, arterial fibrillation and stroke. The ageing heart is exemplified by hypertrophy of tissues and reduction in the potential of the heart rate to respond to a requirement for increase. Given these changes it is very important that the development of other risk factors is minimised. Supporting an older person to eat healthily and exercise will require some understanding of their lifestyle as a younger person. Many men of the 'baby boomer' generation (who are now making up the older generation) will have had sedentary jobs for at least part of their working lives. They may have done sports when younger that they are not able to do now. There is evidence that many men are likely to describe themselves as lonely as they become older (Marmot et al., 2017), and this may be for a number of reasons – loss of contact with work colleagues, death of spouse, divorce, geographical absence of close family members or a lack of established social networks. There is therefore potential for CVD risk factors to develop and add to the physiological risk factors. Nurses working with older people in whatever setting should provide health education – in order to inform about the benefits of a healthy diet and exercise for older people and also in relation to exercise classes or groups that are aimed at older people. Eating smaller amounts of healthy food regularly may suit some older people, and walking a short distance every day can have beneficial effects. One of the most valuable things a nurse can do to support an older man in reducing the risk factors for CVD is to signpost him to social situations or interest groups that might appeal to him.

Secondary prevention of cardiovascular diseases in men

Secondary prevention of CVD in men relates to treating or reducing identified risk factors before they cause irreversible disease. Examples are prescriptions of pharmacological treatments for smoking (nicotine replacement or other products such as varenicline), high blood pressure (from a wide range of antihypertensive medications) or high cholesterol ratio – from a range of statins, or rarely a PCSK9 (proprotein convertase subtilisin/ kexin type 9) inhibitor. This would be accompanied by health education advice, support and signposting to other services in respect of diet, exercise and issues such as stress management if appropriate. A nurse prescriber who issued any of these medications to a patient would do so after determining that there were no existing conditions or treatments that would contraindicate their use and would ensure follow-up appointments were made to assess effectiveness. Attendance at the NHS Health Check would also be part of the process of secondary prevention as it may facilitate early identification of risk factors for CVD and trigger the need for advice and guidance or for medication.

4 Primary and secondary prevention of ill health and health education 2. Children's dental health

Figure 2.4.1 What causes tooth decay?

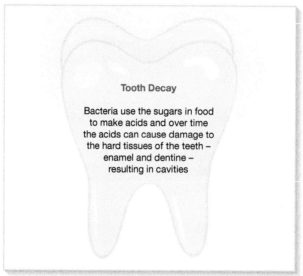

Tooth Decay

Bacteria use the sugars in food to make acids and over time the acids can cause damage to the hard tissues of the teeth – enamel and dentine – resulting in cavities

Figure 2.4.2 Factors that cause tooth decay and gum disease.

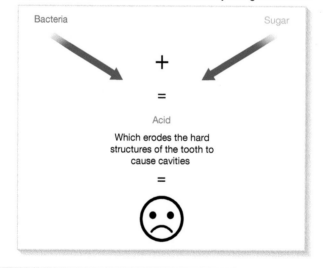

Bacteria

Sugar

+

=

Acid

Which erodes the hard structures of the tooth to cause cavities

=

Children's dental health

The most recent survey on children's oral health reports that 27% of 5-year-olds in England have tooth decay involving 3–4 teeth (Public Health England, 2013). Although the prevalence of tooth decay in children is falling there are still wide geographical variations evident. In the Southeast of England the prevalence of tooth decay is 21.2% of 5-year-olds while in the Northwest the figure is 34.8%. The impact of poor dental health on children's lives can be severe. In addition to the discomfort and pain associated with tooth decay, infection and treatment, loss of primary teeth can impact on speech, eating and appearance. The primary teeth establish space for secondary teeth, which erupt between the ages of 6 and 11 years. Healthy primary teeth allow the secondary teeth to grow and develop normally. If some of the primary teeth are lost early this can lead to overcrowding of dentition and the need to use corrective measures such as braces.

Health protection

One of the health protection measures aimed at reducing tooth decay is the fluoridisation of water supply. Fluoride helps to strengthen and repair tooth enamel making it more resistant to damage from acid attack due to plaque bacteria and sugar. Other health protection measures include the pressures placed by the Food Standards Agency on manufacturers to reduce the amounts of sugar in foodstuffs and the recently announced 'sugar tax' on sugary soft drinks, making them more expensive.

Primary prevention of dental caries

Dental caries is the term used to describe tooth decay resulting from damage to the harder structures of the teeth caused by acids that are produced when the bacteria that form a part of the dental plaque act on sugars in the mouth (Figures 2.4.1 and 2.4.2). Anything that limits the amount of sugar in the mouth and limits build-up of dental plaque will help prevent tooth decay. It is important that children are offered a healthy diet with any sugary foods limited to mealtimes plus inclusion in only one additional snack. Drinks should be of water or milk, and any fruit juices offered should be diluted. Children should drink from a cup or glass as soon as they can safely do so, and any medicines that are required should be sugar-free if possible. These practices all help reduce the amount of sugar in contact with the teeth as well as reducing the duration of contact. In addition it is important that children's teeth are brushed as soon as the primary teeth erupt in order to prevent build-up of the plaque which contains the bacteria involved in tooth decay. Use of a fluoride toothpaste helps to strengthen the enamel of teeth and make them more resistant to decay. Saliva helps neutralise acids produced by plaque bacteria and is very important in dental health. Because saliva production is reduced at night it is important not to offer sugary snacks and drinks to children at bedtime. Some children may be compromised in relation to saliva production – because of medicines being taken, or because they have a condition such as diabetes or a learning disability, or because of a behaviour such as mouth breathing. Particular care should be taken regarding the dental health of these children and wherever possible the situation giving rise to saliva reduction should be addressed.

Clearly these methods of preventing dental caries in children are contingent on parents/carers being aware of them and being able to practise them. Nurses working with children and their families are ideally placed to provide information about preventing tooth decay in children and also to provide support in how to make dental health a practical reality. Parents and carers may need help with ideas of which foodstuffs can replace sugary snacks: options include fruit pieces, vegetable pieces and toast fingers with cheese/or savoury spread. Nurses should be able to advise on how to access affordable healthy foodstuffs, how to store vegetables and fruit for longevity, and where to buy affordable, safe drinking cups. Advice on brushing teeth and supporting children with brushing can be given. Nurses should also signpost families to their nearest dentist and encourage attendance once primary teeth appear. Primary prevention is a combination of advice and practical, realistic, affordable support.

Secondary prevention of dental caries

Secondary prevention aims to limit the progression and impact of early stage dental caries. If slight erosion of tooth enamel is indicated then the dentist can apply fluoride sealants to small fissures to halt the decay. A fluoride varnish can be applied every 4–6 months to the teeth of children deemed at high risk of further dental caries. If caries extends to the dentine layer of the tooth underneath the enamel then an amalgam filling can be used to halt further decay. If the damage to the tooth structure is very severe the tooth may need to be extracted. An average of 3.1% of children aged 5 in England have had one or more teeth extracted, and figures for extraction range from 1.9% in the South-east to 4.6% in Yorkshire and Humber (Public Health England, 2013). An important element of secondary prevention is the offering of the advice and practical support considered under 'Primary prevention'. The dental procedures described are distressing to young children and parents and may involve use of a general anaesthetic. Parents may be more receptive to dental health promotion at this time (see Unit 4) in order to prevent dental caries in their children and avoid further procedures. Nurses should take this opportunity to work with families to enable them to prevent further dental caries in their children and improve family dental health.

Primary and secondary prevention of ill health and health education

3. Self-harm

Figure 2.5.1 Understanding Self Harm. Source: Gateway Counselling Leicester. http://www.gateway-counselling-leicester.co.uk/Cutting-Out-Self-Harm.html.

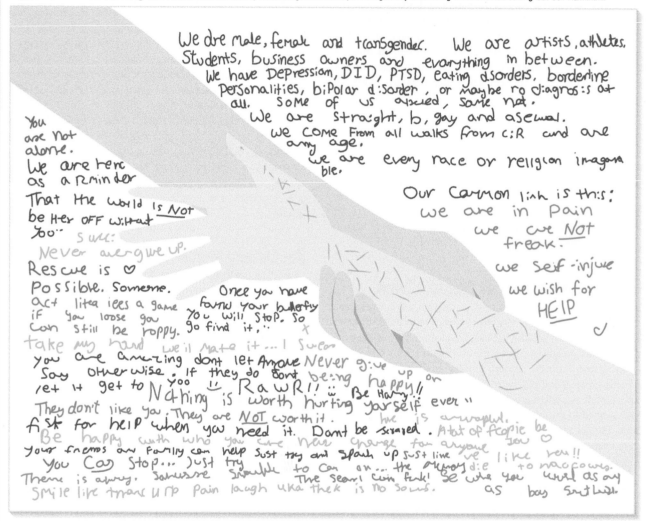

Self-harm

Self-harm is a process by which someone hurts or injures his or herself on purpose rather than by accident. It is the way in which some people deal with overwhelming feelings, memories and emotions that they perceive to be difficult, painful or out of control (Royal College of Psychiatrists, 2017; Mind, 2017a). People of all ages and from all social and cultural backgrounds can perform self-harm (Figure 2.5.1). There is a higher prevalence in prisoners, armed forces veterans, asylum seekers, people who have suffered abuse and neglect as a child, people who use illegal drugs or alcohol and people from sexual minority communities. Hospital episode statistics and results of multi-centre trials suggest that prevalence of self-harm amongst young people is growing, with girls presenting more often than boys. Self-harm can take many different forms including cutting, biting, self-poisoning, overeating or undereating, burning, inserting objects into oneself, hitting oneself, hitting against a surface, excessive exercising, pulling one's own hair, or getting into fights to get hurt.

Primary prevention of self-harm

Because self-harm is a strategy for coping with overwhelming feelings such as desperation, anger, guilt, shame or self-hatred, one aspect of primary prevention is focused on enabling people from a young age to understand different feelings and emotions and what may trigger them as well as learning about strategies that might help in coping with such feelings and emotions. Many schools are teaching pupils about mindfulness techniques or relaxation techniques to help them cope with distressing/frightening feelings and emotions in ways that are not harmful to them. All state schools in the UK are legally required to have a policy in place to identify and prevent bullying, and there is currently a great deal of discussion about how to identify and manage cyber bullying. Because our self-image and self-esteem are largely influenced by the relationships we have with those closest to us, the parent-child relationship and childhood experiences with family and friends can be influential triggers for later self-harming behaviour. Health Visitors, Family Nurse Partnership Nurses and School Health Nurses have important roles to play in identifying poor family interaction and children who lack self-esteem and self-confidence. Attempts can then be made to engage families in learning different ways of behaving towards each other. Strategies can be developed to enable children to have a different image of themselves and their self-worth.

In one sense prevention of self-harming behaviours is everyone's business. Chapter 7 of Unit 1 considered the idea of health-promoting cultures in order to promote best health for all. The ways in which we relate to our families, friends, work colleagues and, as nurses, the patients and clients we meet, need to be positive not negative, encouraging not discouraging, honest and not false. Among the most likely triggers for self-harm are an argument or difficulties in a relationship, and we all have a responsibility to relate to others in ways that acknowledge their right to respect and dignity and that validate their self-worth

Secondary prevention of self-harm

Following an episode of self-harm someone may require medical attention, in which case this should be the first priority before the complex processes of supporting someone to refrain from self-harm begin.

If nurses are working with someone who has self-harmed in any way it is important that they encourage the person to talk and that they listen carefully to try to gain a full picture of the circumstances and events that have led to the episode of self-harm. It is important to remember that self-harm is an indicator that someone has felt overwhelmed by their emotions and feelings. It is not necessarily an indicator of a primary mental health disorder or of an intent to commit suicide. Whilst repeated attempts at self-harm can place someone at higher risk of suicide, many acts of self-harm are perceived by those who carry them out as necessary for survival. Nurses need to listen, respond, encourage and support problem solving in ways that convey that they are authentically present with the patient/client (Watson, 1997).

If a patient wishes to reduce or stop their self-harming behaviour the nurse can support them in three ways (Mind, 2017b).

1 **Understanding their patterns of self-harm.** People can be supported to recognise circumstantial and physiological triggers to self-harm such as a disagreement, an argument, being reminded what a failure they are, a fast heartbeat, sweating, skin flushing, tremors, a feeling of sadness/heaviness/anger, repetitive thoughts – 'I am going to eat all of that' (or cut or skin pick, etc.).

2 **Identify distraction strategies.** Once someone can recognise triggers associated with their self-harming behaviour they can identify actions that might help distract them from harming themselves. These actions are very individual and people should develop what works best for them. (Mind, 2017c).

3 **Delaying self-harm.** For some people, working on delaying the action of self-harm for a period of time can help reduce or stop self-harming episodes. The delay period is a very individual thing and would generally be short, 5–10 minutes. For some people building up the time of delay before self-harming helps over time, and it is also helpful to have someone supporting them with this delay.

Nurses should be aware of the excellent online tools to support people who self-harm as a means of them trying to understand their behaviour, looking after their general health and wellbeing, and receiving support from other people who self-harm currently or who have done in the past. Many people live with self-harming behaviour, and this will be discussed in Chapter 8 of this unit.

Primary and secondary prevention of ill health and health education

4. Obesity and people with a learning disability

Box 2.6.1 Prevention and management of excess weight in people with learning disabilities. Source: Data from Public Health England (2016).

- Use of **appropriate meaningful communication** techniques.
- **Raising awareness** of excess weight in people with learning disabilities and their carers.
- Annual health checks.
- **Support** from families and social care staff.
- **Ensuring accessibility** to mainstream services.
- Environmental, social and personal **barriers**.
- **Capacity and choice** around diet and physical activities.

Public Health and Health Promotion for Nurses at a Glance, First Edition. Karen Wild and Maureen McGrath.
© 2019 John Wiley & Sons Ltd. Published 2019 by John Wiley & Sons Ltd.

Learning disability and obesity

A person is described as having a learning disability if they present with impaired intellect and impaired social functioning that are evident before adulthood and that have a lasting effect on development. They will have a significantly reduced ability to understand new or complex information or to learn new skills and a reduced ability to cope independently (GOV.UK, 2018a). The degree of impairment that someone presents with can be mild, moderate or severe.

People with a learning disability are at increased risk of obesity. This may be due to a poorly balanced diet or a low level of physical activity; people with some conditions, for example Prader–Willi syndrome, will have insatiable appetites making weight management particularly challenging. An important aspect of addressing the health inequalities experienced by people with learning disabilities is enabling them to access either the established services for people with obesity or services tailored to take account of those factors that make such engagement difficult.

There is some evidence that people with a learning disability who are overweight have a much higher rate of those conditions associated with excess weight, such as diabetes, coronary heart disease and cardiovascular disease than the overweight population who do not have a learning disability (GOV.UK, 2018b).

Primary prevention of overweight and obesity in people with a learning disability

Families of babies and young children with a learning disability should follow the same dietary and nutritional advice that all families with children are given. Nurses, health visitors and midwives should be prepared to offer advice and support to families who may be anxious about some of the difficulties that **may** present, such as time taken to complete a feed or difficulties in swallowing. Massaging the cheek gently to stimulate swallowing and working closely with speech and language therapists for additional advice and support are important. As children with a learning disability progress to solid food it is important that they have the same nutritionally balanced diet that is advised for all children. It is important that difficulties around mealtimes do not lead to an approach of letting a child eat when and what they wish in order that they eat something. Again, nurses and health visitors can support families with advice and practical help in this area. There are a number of aids that may help a child who has difficulty with fine or gross motor movements or with some of the sensory skills. Use of plate guards, lipped plates, non-skid plate mats and adapted cutlery may all help when feeding a child or when supporting transition to more independent feeding. If someone eats very slowly it might be important to provide just small amounts of food on the plate at a time so that food can be kept warm and appetising. If someone refuses to eat at mealtimes, just touching the lips gently with a spoon may help. If someone has difficulty chewing then making sure that food is either puréed or cut into small chunks will clearly help.

The point here is that there are lots of pieces of practical advice that might support a family to manage any difficulties around mealtime better (Caroline Walker Trust, 2007). Nurses need to be prepared to model to parents and carers how different advice might be put into practice. It is important that people with a learning disability are encouraged to be as independent as they are realistically and safely able to be as they grow and develop.

Another important aspect of prevention of overweight and obesity is activity and exercise. There are a number of barriers related to the taking of regular exercise by people with a learning disability, including risks to health and safety, transport issues and financial constraints. Learning disability nurses could work alongside people and partner them in some exercise or in attendance at classes. They could also encourage safe exercise within a person's daily routine such as walking or going up and downstairs. It is important to find out what a person really enjoys doing and facilitate their involvement – this may be dancing or drama rather than traditional exercise.

Secondary prevention of overweight and obesity in people with a learning disability

If a person who has a learning disability is overweight there are a number of issues that nurses can take account of to help prevent further weight gain and reduce excess weight (Box 2.6.1). People with a learning disability, in common with everyone else, do not always have an accurate perception of their body mass and shape. There is also some evidence that physical activity is not generally a part of their lives and therefore they remain unaware of its potential physical and mental health benefits. The first thing a nurse may need to do to promote health is to raise awareness of what a healthy weight is. This should be done in an encouraging and positive way. Nurses should also offer their clients an annual health check that looks at lifestyle, medication, health and wellbeing. This can identify particular barriers to healthy diet and activity, and support plans to overcome these can be drawn up. Families and other carers should be aware of and involved in these plans. Support (by nurses or by non-learning-disabled peers) to access mainstream diet and activity groups can provide excellent motivation and can help the experience of attendance to be meaningful and enjoyable. Capacity to make decisions and to maintain safety are important issues for consideration, and again nurses need to relate to people in ways that take account of this but that do not unnecessarily limit opportunities to reduce the risk posed by obesity.

7 Tertiary prevention of ill health and health education: cardiovascular disease in men and dental health in children

Box 2.7.1 Aspects of tertiary prevention of ill health.

All of the work carried out by nurses working with someone at the level of tertiary prevention of ill health should be guided by three principles:
- **This person is very much more than their illness/ condition.**
- **Before you tell, ask.**
- **Do not think 'what condition does this patient have?' but 'what patient does this condition have?'**

The work carried out by nurses working with someone at the level of tertiary prevention of ill health should reflect all of the following:
- Acknowledgement of patient expertise.
- Support to understand the condition and its treatment/ management.
- Facilitation of self-management – of the condition and any medication.
- Signposting to support groups/online support sites.
- Support to recognise change and advice on what to do.
- Coordination of appropriate support services – family and friends, nursing, social care, financial, carer support.
- Health education regarding general health and wellbeing.

Public Health and Health Promotion for Nurses at a Glance, First Edition. Karen Wild and Maureen McGrath.
© 2019 John Wiley & Sons Ltd. Published 2019 by John Wiley & Sons Ltd.

The previous four chapters of this unit have looked at primary and secondary prevention of ill health and associated health education in respect of four different illnesses or conditions. This chapter will consider tertiary prevention in the sense of how nurses might support people to live as well as possible with a long-term illness or condition. There are some guiding principles that should underpin all nurse engagement with patients, and some features that should always be reflected in tertiary prevention work (Box 2.7.1).

Cardiovascular disease (CVD) in men

Nurses supporting a person to live with heart disease or following stroke will need to take time to assess how significantly life has changed for them and to listen to what the person wants, aspires to and fears. Nurses must adopt the attitude that people are the experts in their own lives, and as time progresses will become the experts in living with their condition. Work and leisure activities may be areas that nurses need to discuss with patients in order to practically and realistically consider how someone might return to them or make changes regarding them. People may need support in setting realistic rehabilitation goals for themselves and in being able to carefully monitor and interpret body signals such as pain, fatigue and emotional distress. Cardiac rehabilitation nurses and stroke specialist nurses may also need to be able to support people with advice on general health and wellbeing, sexual health, financial matters and available support groups – both local and online.

The aim of all this work is to enable someone to live the life that they wish to within any constraints that may result from their CVD and to promote general health and wellbeing. Nurses may also work with the immediate family of someone who is living with CVD in order to support their adjustment to any changes and also promote their general health and wellbeing.

Dental caries

Chapter 4 of this unit indicated the importance of good health education to prevent or reduce the development of dental caries in children. The dental health behaviour of the whole family is an important influence on children. If children and young people who already have tooth decay continue to take a lot of sugar in their food and drinks and do not follow recommended dental hygiene practice their teeth may decay to the level when an orthodontic treatment is necessary. This may be because so many primary teeth have been prematurely lost because of decay and this has impacted on the alignment of the secondary teeth. It may be due to secondary teeth having been removed because of decay or needing reconstruction because decay has resulted in cavities that threaten the health of the whole tooth/teeth. These circumstances may mean that a dental prosthetic is required in order to restore dentition and reduce impact on speech, ability to chew and appearance. Examples of prostheses are dental braces, crowns and bridges.

Children and young people who undergo orthodontic procedures will need a lot of support, including age-appropriate discussions about the nature of the procedure, why it is necessary and what the expected result will be. Depending on the procedure they will need to attend the dentist's surgery on several occasions. The procedure may initially impact on the child's appearance in ways that make him/herself conscious and vulnerable to different sorts of bullying. It may well be that dental problems prior to the procedure have impacted on speech or what a child can comfortably eat, and this again may have affected a child's self-esteem and their relationships with others.

Nurses working with children and young people can have a key role in supporting children who are learning to live with the results of dental caries, and their families. This support may include understanding the importance of the prosthetic along with knowledge of how to use it. It should also include support regarding good dental hygiene in order to prevent further procedures. Key aspects of support include strategies to develop self-confidence and self-esteem, both to manage the wearing of the prosthesis and to prevent further caries.

8 Tertiary prevention of ill health and health education: self-harm; obesity in people with a learning disability

---

Box 2.8.1 Aspects of tertiary prevention of ill health.

All of the work carried out by nurses working with someone at the level of tertiary prevention of ill health should be guided by three principles:

- This person is very much more than their illness/condition.
- Before you tell, ask.
- Do not think 'what condition does this patient have?' but 'what patient does this condition have?'

The work carried out by nurses working with someone at the level of tertiary prevention of ill health should reflect all of the following:

- Acknowledgement of patient expertise.
- Support to understand the condition and its treatment/management.
- Facilitation of self-management – of the condition and any medication.
- Signposting to support groups/online support sites.
- Support to recognise change and advice on what to do.
- Coordination of appropriate support services – family and friends, nursing, social care, financial, carer support.
- Health education regarding general health and wellbeing.

Public Health and Health Promotion for Nurses at a Glance, First Edition. Karen Wild and Maureen McGrath.
© 2019 John Wiley & Sons Ltd. Published 2019 by John Wiley & Sons Ltd.

This chapter to continues to look at how nurses can support someone to live well with a long-term condition. It looks at tertiary prevention for people living with self-harm and for people with a learning disability living with obesity. There are some guiding principles that should underpin all nurse engagement with patients, and some features that should always be reflected in tertiary prevention work (Box 2.8.1).

Self-harm

Many people of all ages are living with self-harming behaviour over a long period of time. Nurses supporting someone to live safely within the constraints of their self-harming behaviour tread a very difficult line, and the priority must always be the safety of the person who is self-harming. It is important that nurses equip the people they are working with, and their friends and family if appropriate, to apply principles of both physical and mental health first aid to someone who has harmed themselves. It is important that people are able to recognise when a wound/burn/other injury is serious enough to need immediate medical attention and that they know how to get this. It is also important that friends and family are able to assess the risk of further more serious harm and again how to get help if this is the case.

If an injury can be managed through first aid then people should be aware of how to do this and ensure that relevant dressings and treatments are available. It is also important that people who self-harm have some understanding of their body and the impact of their behaviour on it – this knowledge can, for some people, help contain the behaviour within safe limits. People who self-harm should be encouraged to use professional and other support services such as their GP, community mental health nurses, counsellors and support groups. There are many online resources, and nurses should support people to use those that are safe and well moderated such as the National Self Harm Network (www.nshn.co.uk/), Self-injury Support (www.selfinjurysupport.org.uk/), Selfharm UK (www.selfharm.co.uk//), LifeSIGNS (www.lifesigns.org.uk/), The Mix (www.themix.org.uk/mental-health/self-harm) and SANE (www.sane.org.uk/). Nurses should be aware of the different options available to people who want to treat/disguise/camouflage scars resulting from past self-harm; these include creams and makeup, and the use of tattoos to disguise scars and surgery.

Learning disability and obesity

Some people with a learning disability who are obese will develop one of the conditions associated with obesity such as type 2 diabetes, high blood pressure or a high cholesterol ratio. Supporting a person to live as well as they can with a condition and enabling them to prevent further deterioration of that condition is an important aspect of nursing support. Because of some of the aspects of learning disability described in Chapter 6 of this unit, nurses need to carefully assess the capacity of the person they are working with to give informed consent, understand information and take responsibility for aspects of their condition. For many people with a learning disability they will want a relative or carer to be very involved with managing their condition, and nurses need to be prepared to work in whichever way is preferable.

People should be supported to understand their condition and what it means for them. Given some of the potential cognitive and communication difficulties experienced by some people with a learning disability nurses will need to use appropriate communication techniques such as pictorial explanations of the condition and how best to manage it. It is important to try to present information in clear, concrete and precise ways, and if at all possible to reduce information to one or two key concepts. Nurses should check understanding (and remembering) by asking people to repeat back what they have understood. Using a reminder board or booklet may help someone to consistently manage a condition well. People should be encouraged to manage medication if it is appropriate and safe to do so. Use of dosette boxes and mobile alarm reminders can be helpful in this.

As well as supporting someone to manage their condition nurses need to promote healthy diet and physical activity to prevent further weight gain and slow progression of any obesity-related condition. Some of the aspects considered in Chapter 6 are relevant here, particularly taking care not to offer information overload. The nurse should support a patient/client to overcome barriers to attending mainstream diet and physical activity groups. The University of Sheffield has undertaken a project exploring how best to enable people with a learning disability to access one of the mainstream weight loss organisations, with some initial success (GOV.UK, 2018). Group support can be very important, and some people may wish to access mainstream services while others will want to attend a group tailored specifically to people with a learning disability.

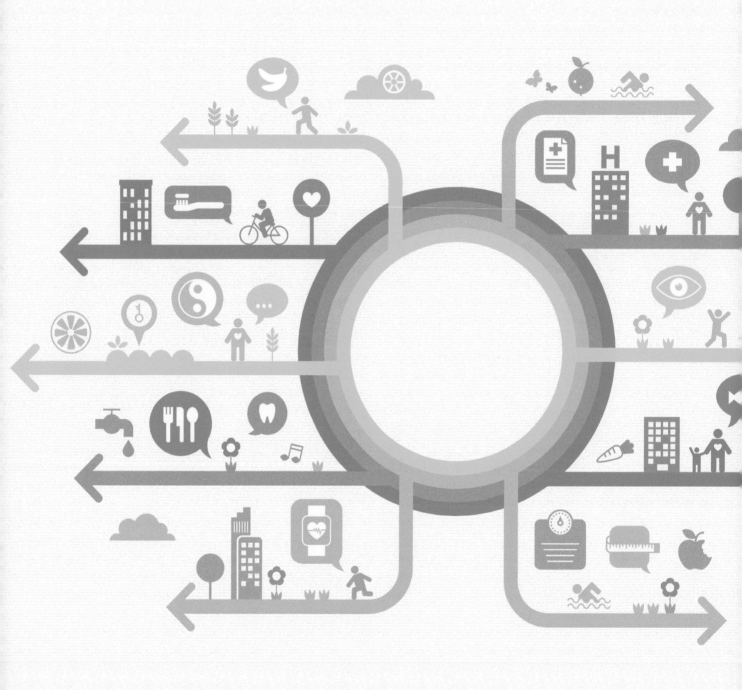

Causes of mortality and morbidity

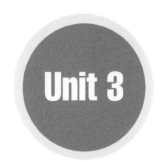

Unit 3

Chapters

Thinking points for NMC Revalidation

In Unit 3 you will gain an understanding of health through the lifespan, which is important in helping nurses to focus on health promotion. What age-related health issues have you encountered in your area of practice and how has health promotion supported those in your care?

1 Different experiences of health through the life course

Box 3.1.1 Elements of wellness. Source: Adapted from Scriven (2010).

- Physical Health – physiological wellbeing, energy, strength, stamina.
- Mental Health – ability to think and discern clearly and coherently.
- Emotional Health – recognition of different emotions (anger, fear, distress) and the ability to express and manage them appropriately.
- Social Health – ability to make and maintain appropriate relationships with family members, friends, neighbours and work colleagues.
- Spiritual Health – discernment of processes, activities, knowledge that promote peace of mind and sense of being at peace with oneself. May relate to faith beliefs but not exclusively.
- Societal Health – relates to legislative, economic and structural society in which we live, at community, national and global levels.

Table 3.1.1 Five ways to wellbeing. Source: Data from Department of Health (2011).

Connect	• Talk to people – face to face • Get to know neighbours, colleagues • Find time to be with other people
Be active	• Do whatever you are able to do may be a little, may be a lot • Do the things that 'light you up'
Take notice	• Take time to look at your environment – wherever you are • Notice what people are wearing, doing, saying without judgement • Notice changes
Keep learning	• Keep on trying new things • Learn a new skill/craft/hobby • Learn about new perspectives from others
Give	• Give your time – to help listen or just be with someone • Know your own abilities and give accordingly • Give spontaneous compliments and acts of kindness

Public Health and Health Promotion for Nurses at a Glance, First Edition. Karen Wild and Maureen McGrath.
© 2019 John Wiley & Sons Ltd. Published 2019 by John Wiley & Sons Ltd.

The life course

The concept of the life course encompasses a number of different ideas. In one sense it is the series of age-related roles and events that people experience in their individual lifetimes as they move though the stages of infancy, childhood, adolescence, young adulthood, midlife and older age. It also acknowledges the different influences of biological, behavioural and psychosocial processes on individuals throughout life and also at particular points in life. It recognises that past and present (and to some extent future) experiences of health are influenced by the wider social, economic and cultural contexts that people experience at different points in their life (World Health Organization, 2000) (Box 3.1.1).

Nurses working with people who are at different stages in the life course should take account of the different ways in which biology, psychology, health behaviours, social relationships and the wider determinants of health (see Chapter 3 in Unit 1) will impact on health, health experience and the process of changing health behaviours.

Experiences of health through the life course

Health experience through the lifespan and changes to health behaviour reflect many of the ideas discussed in Unit 4. Infants and young children are largely dependent on parents/carers in relation to health experience. Older children and adolescents are still influenced by home experiences in relation to health and health behaviours and are also influenced by perceived norms amongst peers and by positive perceptions of negative behaviours represented by all media formats. Infants' and children's early experiences of caregiving and of structure and stability impact on their emotional and psychological development in relation to self-efficacy, resilience and ability to form satisfactory relationships with others, all of which will impact on health experiences. As well as home influences children and young people are subject to an increasing number of positive and negative influences through traditional and social media, and it is important that services aimed at this age group recognise and respond to this.

Young adults are more independent in terms of their health behaviours and are generally thought to be more likely to experiment with risky health behaviours (as are adolescents). Young adults living in the UK in the twenty-first century can also feel under considerable pressures in relation to education, employment and the opportunity to live independently of parents/carers as the nature of work and the emphasis placed on educational achievement has altered considerably over the last 10–20 years. Adult health behaviour is influenced by employment (and stability of employment), educational achievement, income, relationship and family responsibilities – both for younger and older family members, work environment, neighbourhood environment and opportunities for leisure activities. The latter can be compromised by lack of time, lack of money or availability of anyone to enjoy leisure time with. Older people's health experiences will be influenced by biological health status. Many older people are fit and healthy into advanced old age. However, ageing does result in changes to body systems such as the cardiovascular, immune and endocrine systems, and many people will experience disease processes related to the musculoskeletal system. Many people experience loneliness in old age (Age UK, 2014). Ageing is a very individual process and we are learning more about the individual genetic control of cellular ageing. Hence it is important that nurses working to promote health in older people take time to get to know the individual abilities, frailties, wishes and intentions of their clients/patients.

Readiness to change through the life course

Research looking at health behaviours through the life course has identified six self-reported behaviours that may negatively impact on health (Williams et al., 2012). These are nutrition, physical activity, smoking, alcohol consumption, drug use and unprotected sex. In this report nearly every adult reported at least one negative health behaviour, and one-fifth of adults reported three or more negative behaviours. The report identified times in the life course that seemed to trigger a readiness to engage in behaviour change. These were moving in with a partner, becoming a parent (though the researchers indicate that changed behaviour may not necessarily be sustained) and getting older. The research indicated that those who engage in risk behaviours such as smoking and drug use appear to reduce these behaviours in the mid-thirties age group, and a government report published in 2014 has suggested that risk behaviours and outcomes such as smoking, alcohol/drug use and teenage pregnancy have steadily declined in the under-25 age group over the last decade (HM Government, 2014). There is evidence that the incidence of sexually transmitted diseases is rising in older adults (over 50) and that harmful drinking is an issue for between 10 and 20% of older people.

The health behaviours of adults will directly impact on the health of children and young adults. For all age groups in the research of Williams et al. (2012) the negative health behaviours that were most prevalent were poor nutrition (measured as consuming less than five portions of fruit and vegetables daily) and lack of physical activity (less than 150 minutes of cardiovascular activity). This is reflected in the increasing prevalence of obesity in the UK (with the exception of Ireland and Northern Ireland), which impacts on both physical and mental wellbeing for all age groups.

It is important that factors that impact on mental health and wellbeing through the life course are taken into account by nurses working with patients at the different stages of life. The patterns of life experienced by many people in the twenty-first century can pose a threat to health in terms of stress, anxiety, perception of self-esteem and self-efficacy for many of the reasons mentioned above. Nurses should model the five ways to wellbeing (Table 3.1.1) and also encourage their patients/clients to be aware of them and practise them.

2 Long-term conditions: all ages

Table 3.2.1 Proportion of people with long-term conditions (LTCs) by age in England. Source: Department of Health (2012). Licensed under Open Government Licence v3.0. http://www.nationalarchives.gov.uk/doc/open-government-licence/version/3/).

Age Group	Percentage of people with a long term condition
0–9	10%
10–19	12%
20–29	17%
30–39	20%
40–49	27%
50–59	40%
60–69	52%
70–79	63%
80 +	70%

Table 3.2.2 Most prevalent long-term conditions (LTCs). Source: Department of Health (2012). Licensed under Open Government Licence v3.0. http://www.nationalarchives.gov.uk/doc/open-government-licence/version/3/.

Adults	• Hypertension • Depression • Asthma
Conditions rising most quickly are	• Cancers • Chronic kidney disease • Diabetes • Dementia
Some LTCs are not included in QoF disease registers	• Some musculoskeletal conditions
Children	• Diabetes • Asthma • Epilepsy • Allergies

Public Health and Health Promotion for Nurses at a Glance, First Edition. Karen Wild and Maureen McGrath.

Long-term conditions

A long term condition (LTC) is a condition that cannot at present be cured but is controlled by medication and/or other treatments/therapies (Department of Health, 2012). Long-term conditions can affect children and adults of all ages but prevalence increases with age (Table 3.2.1). Long-term illness may be primarily a physical or mental health condition but it is common for someone who is living with a LTC to have both mental and physical comorbidities. Long-term conditions are increasing in prevalence. They may have considerable impact on attendance at work or school and also on social and economic capital. People from lower socioeconomic groups have a greater risk of developing a LTC.

Long-term conditions are thought to account for:

- 50% of all GP appointments
- 64% of all outpatient appointments
- 70% of all inpatient bed days
- 70% of the total health and social care budget.

The most prevalent LTCs in adults and children are shown in Table 3.2.2.

How nurses can support people living with LTCs

All research into the best ways of enabling people to live with LTCs (Department of Health, 2012, 2013; The King's Fund, 2012; NHS England, 2017) emphasises that maximising self-management of the condition, promoting shared decision making and enabling choice should underpin any and all of the engagement that health professionals have with patients in these circumstances.

One of the most important things a nurse can do is to actively listen to the patient and their family/carers. Patients who are living with a LTC should be seen as the experts in their condition and how it impacts on their lives. Nurses need to be able to assess very clearly what needs the person has and then support them in problem solving and accessing resources in order to address those needs. Patients should always be involved in making any decision about their support and care, and nurses can enable this through providing more information about their condition and about the resources and different types of care available to them. People with a LTC may need support to develop self-confidence and self-efficacy in managing their condition, and nurses can draw on some of the skills mentioned in Unit 4, Chapters 4, 5 and 6, in helping them to develop these skills.

One aspect of care that people with LTCs consistently mention is that they wish to avoid hospitalisation unless absolutely necessary, and that they wish to work with services in a proactive way to facilitate a planned approach to any necessary hospitalisation and avoid emergency admissions. Nurses need to be involved in providing support that coordinates the different health and social care support services that may be working with someone with a LTC. People want joined up seamless services that act as one team. As indicated above many people who have LTCs will be living with both mental and physical comorbidities, and 20% of people with an LTC describe themselves as living with three or more conditions. This can result in a number of very complex needs, and it is important that these are not considered and addressed in isolation and that there is recognition of the ways in which the different conditions all impact on each other to create needs for the individual. People with one or more conditions wish to be treated as a whole person.

People with a LTC may go through a series of transitions as their condition develops, which may involve loss of function, increased medication and greater difficulties in self-managing their condition. For children living with a LTC they will also undergo the transitions involved in developing into adulthood and the accompanying changes in service provision. Nurses can have a key role in recognising the potential for these transitions and ensuring that people are prepared for possible changes. Service coordination is essential, and a move to joint commissioning and closer working between health and social care services could make a real difference to people with a LTC who wish to plan how they will manage these transitions.

Nurses need to be mindful of the needs of the carers of people living with a LTC. These are usually family members and include young carers (aged 18 or under). All carers whatever their age have a right to a needs assessment by the local authority, and nurses must ensure that they are aware of this. The health of a person with LTC and the health of their carer/s are closely linked, and part of the nurse's role in supporting a patient is to engage with their carer to promote their health and wellbeing also.

One of the most helpful experiences for people is to learn about how people with the same LTC have developed the skills to confidently self-manage their condition and associated medications and treatments. Nurses should be familiar with local and online support groups that are credible and that can provide this opportunity.

The nurse has a role in promoting health in a wider sense with people who live with a LTC and their families/carers. As well as enabling someone to confidently self-manage their condition and be prepared for any health transitions, nurses can promote general health and wellbeing in relation to nutrition and physical activity (within the constraints the LTC imposes). Nurses can also assess someone's readiness to discuss other health issues such as smoking, use of drugs or alcohol and sexual wellbeing. Promotion of mental wellbeing through use of the five ways to mental wellbeing mentioned in Chapter 1 of this unit and through strategies such as meditation, mindfulness or counselling may also be helpful following careful assessment of need.

3 Cardiovascular diseases

Figure 3.3.1 Risk factor for cardiovascular disease: high blood pressure (BP). Source: Public Health England. Licensed under Open Government Licence v3.0. http://www.nationalarchives.gov.uk/doc/open-government-licence/version/3/.

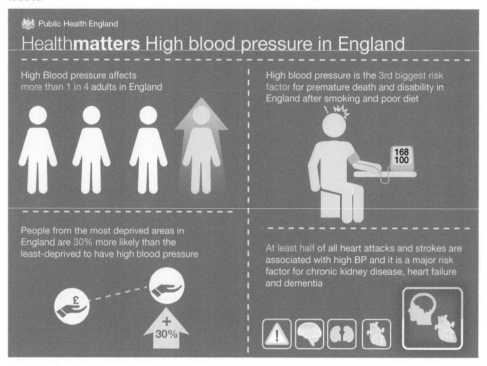

Figure 3.3.2 Screening for hypertension: the NHS Health Check. Source: National Health Service. Licensed under Open Government Licence v3.0. http://www.nationalarchives.gov.uk/doc/open-government-licence/version/3/.

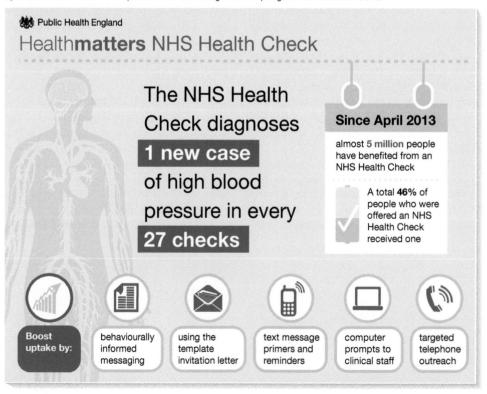

Introduction

Cardiovascular disease (CVD) is an umbrella term that describes all diseases of the heart and circulation. It includes everything from conditions that are diagnosed at birth, or inherited, to developed conditions such as coronary heart disease, atrial fibrillation, heart failure and stroke. According to the British Heart Foundation (2018):

- Cardiovascular (heart and circulatory) disease causes more than a quarter (26%) of all deaths in the UK; that's nearly 160 000 deaths each year – an average of 435 people each day or one death every three minutes.
- Around 42 000 people under the age of 75 in the UK die from CVD each year.
- Since the BHF was established the annual number of deaths from CVD in the UK has fallen by half.
- In 1961, more than half of all deaths in the UK were attributed to CVD (320 000 CVD deaths).
- Since 1961 the UK death rate from CVD has declined by more than three-quarters. Death rates have fallen more quickly than the actual number of deaths because people in this country are now living longer lives.

Risk factors

Many different risk factors increase an individual's likelihood of developing CVD (Figure 3.3.1):

- Nearly 30% of adults in the UK have hypertension.
- High blood cholesterol is a significant risk factor.
- Having diabetes can double the risk of developing CVD (3.6 million adults in the UK have been diagnosed with diabetes).
- In the UK around 10% of those diagnosed are living with type 1 diabetes and 90% have type 2, with an estimated 1 million who are undiagnosed.

Modifiable risk factors (e.g. cigarette smoking, physical inactivity and poor diet) contribute significantly to the risk of CVD:

- More than one in six adults smoke cigarettes in the UK – that's around 9 million adults.
- Nearly 100 000 smokers in the UK die from smoking-related causes each year.
- Each year an estimated 20 000 UK deaths from CVD can be attributed to smoking.
- Over one-quarter (27%) of adults in the UK are obese, and more than one-third are overweight (by BMI).

It is estimated that nearly 30% of children in the UK are overweight or obese. Nearly two out of five adults in the UK do not achieve recommended levels of physical activity.

- Only one-quarter of UK adults and one in five children eat the recommended minimum portions of fruit and vegetables per day.
- One-quarter of adults in the UK exceed national guidelines for weekly alcohol intake; no level of use is without risk.

Other risk factors can significantly increase the risk of developing CVD include age, gender, family history and ethnicity.

Hypertension – the silent killer

After smoking and poor diet, hypertension is the third biggest risk factor in CVD. It affects more than one in four adults in England. Seldom causing symptoms, hypertension has been hailed as the 'silent killer'. It is also recognised as the biggest risk factor for stroke.

- The National Institute for Health and Care Excellence (NICE) defines high blood pressure, also known as hypertension, as a clinic blood pressure of 140/90 mmHg or higher and either a subsequent ambulatory blood pressure monitoring daytime average or home blood pressure monitoring average of 135/85 mmHg or higher.
- Blood pressure readings between 120/80 and 140/90 mmHg are defined as high normal blood pressure. High blood pressure doesn't just happen to older adults. Over 2.1 million people under the age of 45 had high blood pressure in England in 2015 (PHE, 2017).

Make every contact count

Improving the prevention, detection and management of hypertension is an important nursing role. Opportunities to engage in health promotion and education in relation to high blood pressure are equally important when supporting individuals with long-term health problems, or within routine screening activities such as the NHS Health Check (Figure 3.3.2).

When engaging with patients and clients:

- Discuss healthy lifestyles and modifiable risk factors to aid the prevention of hypertension.
- Carefully screen for the presence of hypertension.
- Highlight the national ACT FAST campaign to raise awareness of the common symptoms of stroke and what to do in an emergency.
- Download resources from the British Heart Foundation (BHF) (https://www.bhf.org.uk/healthcare-professionals/commissioning-and-services/service-innovation/bp-how-can-we-do-better).

4 Respiratory diseases

Figure 3.4.1 Deaths each year from chronic obstructive pulmonary disease (COPD) in the UK. Source: British Lung Foundation (2016). Reproduced with permission of the British Lung Foundation.

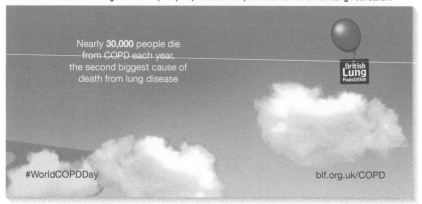

Nearly **30,000** people die from COPD each year, the second biggest cause of death from lung disease

British Lung Foundation

#WorldCOPDDay

blf.org.uk/COPD

Figure 3.4.2 Attempts and success at quitting smoking. Source: Public Health England. Licensed under Open Government Licence v3.0. http://www.nationalarchives.gov.uk/doc/open-government-licence/version/3/.

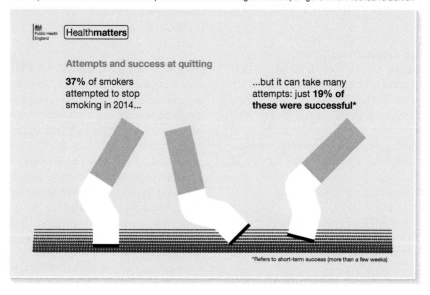

Public Health England

Health**matters**

Attempts and success at quitting

37% of smokers attempted to stop smoking in 2014...

...but it can take many attempts: just **19% of these were successful***

*Refers to short-term success (more than a few weeks)

Introduction

The British Heart Foundation (BHF) regularly reports on the most recent statistics that relate to respiratory disease in the UK. Some 12.7 million people in the UK (i.e. one in five people) have a history of asthmah chronic obstructive pulmonary disorder (COPD) or another longstanding respiratory illness. Around half of these people are taking prescribed medicines for lung disease. Estimates based on general practice records suggest that 8 million people have been diagnosed with asthma, 1.2 million with COPD and over 150 000 with interstitial lung diseases (pulmonary or sarcoidosis), with numbers generally similar for males and females. GP records suggest there are over 32 000 new cases of lung cancer and over 2000 new cases of mesothelioma annually (ONS, 3).

During 2008–2012, lung diseases were responsible for 20% of all deaths in the UK annually. This figure has seen little change, unlike cardiovascular diseases where the proportion of deaths has declined: the proportion due to lung diseases has remained constant.

Over half the deaths from lung disease in the UK are due to lung cancer and COPD (Figure 3.4.1 shows deaths from COPD). Both conditions are strongly linked to tobacco smoking, which is also a risk factor for pneumonia, another leading cause of death. In 2012, 6.2% of all UK deaths were due to lung cancer, 5.3% to COPD and 5.1% to pneumonia (ONS, 3).

Risk factors

By far the most fundamental risk factor for all respiratory diseases in the UK is cigarette smoking.
- Smoking is the main cause of COPD and is thought to be responsible for four out of every five cases.
- Individuals are more likely to develop COPD if they smoke and have a close relative with the condition, suggesting some people's genes may make them more vulnerable to the condition.
- Exposure to certain types of dust and chemicals at work may damage the lungs and increase the risk of COPD. Substances that have been linked to COPD include:
  - cadmium dust and fumes
  - grain and flour dust
  - silica dust
  - welding fumes
  - isocyanates
  - coal dust.

- Tobacco smoking and environmental tobacco smoke (ETS, also called second-hand smoke) are classified by the International Agency for Research on Cancer (IARC) as causes of lung cancer. An estimated 86% of lung cancers in the UK are linked to tobacco smoking – 83% due to active smoking, and 3% due to ETS exposure in non-smokers.
- Exposure to air pollution over a long period can affect how well the lungs work, and some research has suggested it could increase your risk of COPD. At the moment the link between air pollution and COPD isn't conclusive and research is continuing.
- Diet and nutrition.
- Postinfectious chronic respiratory diseases.

Making every contact count

Nurses play a significant part in raising the awareness of respiratory health issues and influencing local and national health care policy. Interventions can include supporting initiatives such as the Cold Weather Plan and the Heatwave Plan, identifying groups and associated agencies who may be at risk.

Other examples of health promotion interventions include:
- Supporting patients to quit smoking through direct action and referral. Figure 3.4.2 highlights the potential success rates following attempts to quit smoking.
- Supporting the uptake of flu and pneumonia vaccinations to reduce complications and avoidable hospital admissions (also individual).
- Referring patients to pulmonary rehabilitation when appropriate; this is a treatment that has been shown to reduce admissions, improve exercise capacity and improve quality of life.
- Support postdischarge to ensure patients who have been admitted to hospital with an exacerbation of COPD or an asthma attack are given support by the appropriate health-care professional to prevent readmissions.

Nurses can have an impact on an individual level by:
- Following NICE guidelines when providing advice and support for smoking cessation. Visit the NHS SMOKEFREE website with your patients and clients.
- Providing a personalised action plan for all patients as these reduce readmission rates, increase patient wellbeing and reduce frequency of attacks.
- Promoting and checking inhaler techniques in ill children and adults on an annual basis.

5 Cancers

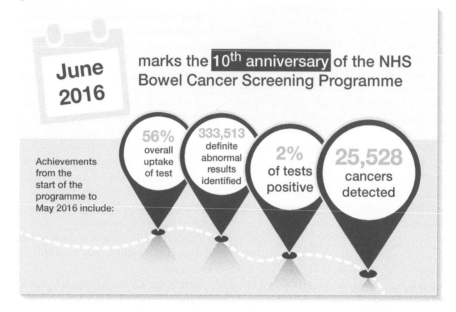

Figure 3.5.1 Achievements in the UK Bowel Cancer Screening Programme. Source: Public Health England. Licensed under Open Government Licence v3.0. http://www.nationalarchives.gov.uk/doc/open-government-licence/version/3/.

June 2016 marks the 10th anniversary of the NHS Bowel Cancer Screening Programme

Achievements from the start of the programme to May 2016 include:

56% overall uptake of test

333,513 definite abnormal results identified

2% of tests positive

25,528 cancers detected

Figure 3.5.2 Smoking and cancer. Source: National Health Service. Licensed under Open Government Licence v3.0. http://www.nationalarchives.gov.uk/doc/open-government-licence/version/3/.

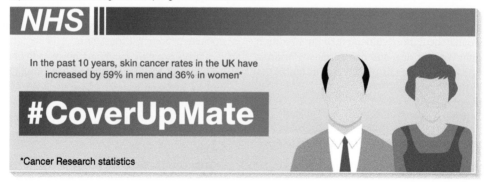

NHS

In the past 10 years, skin cancer rates in the UK have increased by 59% in men and 36% in women*

#CoverUpMate

*Cancer Research statistics

Introduction

According to Cancer UK, more than one in two people will develop cancer at some point in their lives. Every year more than 350 000 people are diagnosed with the disease. This places nurses in a prime position to engage in education and prevention to reduce the incidence of cancer and support those who are at risk or suffering from the effects of cancer.

Experts predict that more than four in ten cases of cancer could be prevented, largely through lifestyle changes that include not smoking, maintaining a healthy body weight, eating healthily, reducing alcohol intake, protecting skin from the sun and keeping active. In addition, nurses can be instrumental in supporting people to avoid infections such as human papillomavirus (HPV) or hepatitis and to be safe within the workplace when exposed to dangerous risks.

Risk factors

Smoking – this is the biggest risk factor, with smoking accounting for one in four UK cancer deaths and almost one-fifth of all cancer cases. Smoking represents the biggest avoidable risk factor in cancer.

Alcohol is one of the most established risk factors associated with cancer. The types of cancer most associated with alcohol include mouth and upper throat cancers and cancer of the bowel. Alcohol is also associated with breast and liver cancer. One theory that aligns with the evidence is that alcohol affects DNA. Alcohol when digested is converted into acetaldehyde, which can cause cancer by damaging DNA and preventing it from being repaired.

Diet can potentiate cancer in a number of ways. Maintaining a healthy body weight significantly reduces the risk of cancers. Diets that are high in salt and low in dietary fibre are implicated in stomach and bowel cancer. Processed and red meats are also implicated in the incidence of bowel cancer. Figure 3.5.1 highlights the success of bowel screening to detect lower bowel cancers in the UK. Eating a diet that is rich in fruit and vegetables supports immunity and reduces obesity.

Obesity is the second most effective modifiable risk factor in preventing cancer. A recent report by Cancer Research UK and the UK Health Forum (2016) predicts that by 2035 three in four adults will be overweight or obese if current trends continue.

This could lead to an extra 670 000 cases of cancer in the UK over the next 20 years.

Inactivity can lead to such conditions as obesity, type 2 diabetes and cardiovascular problems. It is also linked to the associated risks of cancer of the bowel and breast.

The sun and UV light. Overexposure to ultraviolet (UV) light from the sun or sun beds is the main cause of skin cancer. Some people are more likely than others to develop skin cancer. These people tend to have one or more of the following: Fair skin that burns easily in the sun, an abundance of moles and freckles, a history of sunburn, fair or red hair and light coloured eyes, and a family history of skin cancer. Figure 3.5.2 highlights the move to create more awareness of skin cancer in men in England.

Infections such as HPV, *Helicobacter* and HIV can increase the risk of cancers if left untreated. People can't **catch** cancer, but acquiring infections through lifestyle choices can increase risk.

Environmental pollutants are beginning to be researched more closely to establish the links between air pollution and cancer. Early research suggests that the links are real.

Occupational risk is related to exposure; for example, manufacturing workers exposed to silica, asbestos or solvents, or those in the service industry exposed to exhaust fumes.

Making every contact count

Most commonly as a nurse in practice, a lifestyle issue will be about encouraging individuals to:

- stop smoking
- eat healthily
- maintain a healthy weight
- drink alcohol within the recommended daily limits
- undertake the recommended amount of physical activity
- avoid potentially harmful environments and raise awareness about risks associated with pollutants and occupational harms.

Communications that have true meaning will put the focus on the individual and their needs. A therapeutic relationship that is mutual and genuine will enable a more open approach to discussions and interventions around lifestyle areas such as sexual health or being immunised. It may also involve ensuring individuals can access services to support the wider determinants of health, such as housing or financial support, which may be barriers to making a healthy lifestyle choice.

6 Child and adolescent mental health

Figure 3.6.1 The incidence of childhood and adolescent mental health problems. Source: https://www.mentalhealth.org.uk/statistics/mental-health-statistics-children-and-young-people. Reproduced with permission of Mental Health Foundation.

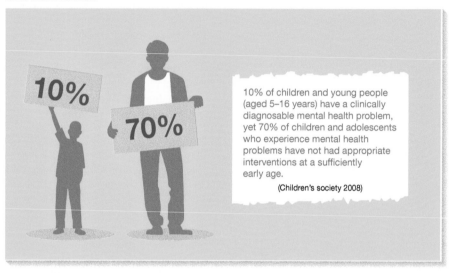

10% of children and young people (aged 5–16 years) have a clinically diagnosable mental health problem, yet 70% of children and adolescents who experience mental health problems have not had appropriate interventions at a sufficiently early age.

(Children's society 2008)

Figure 3.6.2 Websites that support childhood and adolescent mental heath.

'Place2Be'
- A charity that provides emotional and therapeutic services to children and young people in school, supporting them to cope with complex social issues such as bullying, death, violence and abuse, family breakdown
- www.place2be.org.uk

'The Mix'
- This is the UK's leading support service for young people, offering a wide range of advice and help. Included in the support is information and help with regard to mental health issues and drug abuse
- www.themix.org.uk

'Young minds'
- The UK's leading charity championing the wellbeing and mental health of young people, from Government policy to practice in schools and services. It supports parents to help their children through difficult times, and equips professionals to provide the best possible support to the young people that they work with, empowering young people to change their world
- www.youngminds.org.uk

'Best Beginnings'
- The aim here is to support families in giving children the best start in life
- www.bestbeginnings.org.uk

Public Health and Health Promotion for Nurses at a Glance, First Edition. Karen Wild and Maureen McGrath.
© 2019 John Wiley & Sons Ltd. Published 2019 by John Wiley & Sons Ltd.

Introduction

The majority of young people grow and develop being mentally healthy. Over decades, experiences of growing up have changed, and there is a growing body of research that suggests that more children and young people are suffering from mental health problems today compared with 30 years ago. Caring for a young person's emotional wellbeing is just as important as caring for their physical wellbeing. Figure 3.6.1 shows that an estimated one in ten children and young people in the UK are affected by mental health problem, and 70% of these have not received suitable intervention and help at an early age. The key problems centre on depression, anxiety and behavioural problems, many of which are as a direct result of a young person's social environment.

• Depression is more likely to be seen in teenagers than young children. The number of young people aged between 15 and 16 with depression nearly doubled between the 1980s and the 2000s (Nuffield Foundation, 2013).

• Self-harm can be a way of managing deep emotional pain. Cutting and burning are, and self-harm affects around 1 in 12 people, with 10% of 12–15-year-olds self-harming (https://youngminds.org.uk/).

• Generalised anxiety disorder (GAD) can occur, for example, when young people worry excessively about change or separation from their peer group.

• Post-traumatic stress disorder (PTSD) can occur as a reaction to exposure to events, abuse, trauma, bullying, etc.

• Attention deficit hyperactivity disorder (ADHD) is where children show little ability to concentrate and behave in an unexpected or compulsive manner. More common in males than females.

• Eating disorders, such as bulimia and anorexia nervosa, can commonly start in adolescence and are seen more in females than males.

• Suicide remains a leading cause of death in young people in the UK. In England 149 children between 10 and 19 years of age committed suicide in 2014 – almost three children every week (Korkodilos, 2016).

Recent campaigns to highlight the issue and to promote better understanding of the stigma and incidence of mental health have been championed by the Duke and Duchess of Cambridge and Prince Harry. The focus of their work is to help young people to speak out about mental health issues and to engage the public in talking more openly about the subject. The Heads Together initiative will work with other charities to support the aims (www.headstogether.org.uk).

Risk factors

A number of risk factors can be linked to the incidence of mental health problems in young people. They include:

• Poor physical health
• Poor nutrition
• Long-term illness
• History of mental illness in parents
• Alcohol misuse within the family
• Parents with criminal history
• Loss and bereavement
• Bullying, abuse, discrimination
• Separation or divorce of parents
• Homelessness, poverty
• Carer responsibilities
• Learning difficulties.

Making every contact count

School nursing teams provide vital services for children and young people. A recent survey carried out on behalf of the Children's Commissioner for England (2016) demonstrated that school nurses are ideally placed to provide the accessible, non-stigmatised advice that children and young people need as part of everyday life.

Children and Young People's mental health nurses have a key role in providing direct support to children, young people and their families. In addition they can educate and support other professionals to promote emotional and psychological wellbeing in young people. Timely and appropriate access to health care can make all the difference to a child's long-term health and wellbeing, with interventions such as cognitive behavioural therapy, dialectical therapy and family therapy, as well as the management of deliberate self-harm.

MindEd is a free educational resource jointly funded by the Departments of Health and Education. It aims to coach professionals, as well as parents and carers. There are two resources:

• MindEd for Families – online advice and information to help families understand and identify early issues and how best to support children. Specific pathways have been developed to signpost school nurses and others to key modules to complete.

• MindEd for Professionals and Volunteers – provides adults who care or work with young people with the knowledge to support their wellbeing, the understanding to identify a child at risk of a mental health condition, and the confidence to act on their concern and, if needed, signpost to services that can help (www.minded.org.uk).

Figure 3.6.2 shows resources that nurses can access or refer to others.

7 Depression

> **Box 3.7.1** National Institute for Health and Care Excellence (NICE) guidance for dealing with depression in adults: providing information and support, and obtaining informed consent. Source: Data from NICE (2016).
>
> When working with people with depression and their families or carers:
> - Build a trusting relationship and work in an open, engaging and non-judgemental manner.
> - Explore treatment options in an atmosphere of hope and optimism, explaining the different courses of depression and that recovery is possible.
> - Be aware that stigma and discrimination can be associated with a diagnosis of depression.
> - Ensure that discussions take place in settings in which confidentiality, privacy and dignity are respected.
>
> When working with people with depression and their families or carers:
> - Provide information appropriate to their level of understanding about the nature of depression and the range of treatments available.
> - Avoid clinical language without adequate explanation.
> - Ensure that comprehensive written information is available in the appropriate language and in audio format if possible.
> - Provide and work proficiently with independent interpreters (i.e. someone who is not known to the person with depression) if needed.
>
> Inform people with depression about self-help groups, support groups and other local and national resources.
> Make all efforts necessary to ensure that a person with depression can give meaningful and informed consent before treatment starts. This is especially important when a person has severe depression or is subject to the Mental Health Act.
>
> Ensure that consent to treatment is based on the provision of clear information (which should also be available in written form) about the intervention, covering:
> - what it comprises
> - what is expected of the person while having it
> - likely outcomes (including any side effects).

Public Health and Health Promotion for Nurses at a Glance, First Edition. Karen Wild and Maureen McGrath.
© 2019 John Wiley & Sons Ltd. Published 2019 by John Wiley & Sons Ltd.

Introduction

Depression is characterised by persistent low mood, which may present as a loss of pleasure in most activities. Typically people who are depressed convey a range of associated emotional, cognitive, physical and behavioural symptoms. The incidence of depression amongst the population is surprisingly high, and nurses are extremely likely to care for and support individuals who are suffering. Within the primary care setting, depression is the third most common GP consultation, with around 1 in 20 adults experiencing a period of depression; on average a person may suffer for 6–8 months.

In 2016 the Office for National Statistics report 'Measuring national well-being: Life in the UK' highlighted that some evidence of anxiety or depression, according to the General Health Questionnaire (GHQ-12), increased to 19.7%, from 18.3% in the previous year. Mental health is a factor that affects wellbeing. The report went on to state that:

> People with positive mental health will feel good about themselves, and will feel they are better equipped to cope with their problems, whereas those people that indicate depression or anxiety may find this more challenging. This will undoubtedly impact on personal and therefore national well-being.
>
> ONS (2016)

Risk factors

There are a number of stresses contributing to the development of depression; these can include:

- Worries with finance or employment.
- Problems with interpersonal relationships.
- Poor living conditions.
- Bereavement and major depression share many symptoms, but active suicidal thoughts, psychotic symptoms and profound guilt are rare with normal bereavement.
- A personal and family history of depression.

The risk of recurrence is at least 50% after a first episode of depression, 70% after a second episode and 90% after a third episode. This is increased in people under 20 years of age, and in elderly people.

Make every contact count

Nurses should be aware of the symptoms of depression when engaging in therapeutic relationships. Typical symptoms include:

- Feeling down, depressed or hopeless ('core' symptom).
- Little interest or pleasure in doing things ('core' symptom).
- Fatigue/loss of energy.
- Worthlessness/excessive or inappropriate guilt.
- Recurrent thoughts of death, suicidal thoughts or actual suicide attempts.
- Diminished ability to think/concentrate or indecisiveness.
- Psychomotor agitation or retardation.
- Insomnia/hypersomnia.
- Significant appetite and/or weight loss.
- Reactive mood, increased appetite, weight gain, excessive sleepiness and sensitivity to rejection.

The National Institute for Health and Care Excellence (NICE, 2016) provides comprehensive guidelines to support practitioners in their interactions with people who suffer from depression. Box 3.7.1 outlines activities that the nurse and practitioners should engage in when supporting patients who are depressed and their families and carers.

Nurses can actively screen people who are at high risk (e.g. those with a history of depression, or significant physical illness). Ask about the two 'core' symptoms of depression:

- During the last month have you often been bothered by feeling down, depressed or hopeless?
- Do you have little interest or pleasure in doing things?

If the answer to these questions is 'Yes', then a referral to a mental health practitioner is recommended. Depression can be assessed using a range of tools, which often relate to the *Diagnostic and Statistical Manual of Mental Disorders Fifth Edition* (DSM-5) classification by the presence of at least five out of a possible nine defining symptoms, present for at least 2 weeks, of sufficient severity to cause clinically significant distress or impairment in social, occupational or other important areas of functioning (American Psychiatric Association, 2013).

People with depression should be assessed and managed for the risk of suicide, the associated safeguarding risks if there are children or vulnerable others involved, and the conditions associated with depression. Conditions associated with depression include anxiety, alcohol or substance abuse, eating disorders, psychotic symptoms and dementia.

8 Dementia

Table 3.8.1 Risk factors associated with dementia. Source: Data from The Alzheimer's Society (2014).

Risk factor	Rationale
Age	The chances of developing dementia rise significantly as we get older. Above the age of 65, a person's risk of developing Alzheimer's disease or vascular dementia doubles roughly every 5 years. In addition other associated reasons include loss of sex hormones and reduced immunity with aging
Gender	Women are more likely to develop Alzheimer's disease than men. For most dementias other than Alzheimer's disease, men and women have much the same risk. For vascular dementia, men are actually at slightly higher risk than women. This is because men are more prone to stroke and heart disease, which can cause vascular and mixed dementia
Genetics	More than 20 genes have been found that do not directly cause dementia but affect a person's risk of developing it. For example, inheriting certain versions (variants) of the gene apolipoprotein E (APOE) increases a person's risk of developing Alzheimer's disease. Having a close relative (parent or sibling) with Alzheimer's disease increases your own chances of developing the disease very slightly compared to someone with no family history It is also possible to inherit genes that directly cause dementia, although these are much rarer than the risk genes like APOE. In affected families there is a very clear pattern of inheritance of dementia from one generation to the next. This pattern is seen in families with familial Alzheimer's disease (a very rare form of Alzheimer's that appears usually well before the age of 60) and genetic frontotemporal dementia
Ethnicity	There is some evidence that people from certain ethnic communities are at higher risk of dementia than others. For example, South Asian people (from countries such as India and Pakistan) seem to develop dementia – particularly vascular dementia – more often than white Europeans. South Asians are well known to be at a higher risk of stroke, heart disease and diabetes, and this is thought to explain the higher dementia risk. Similarly, people of African or African-Caribbean origin seem to develop dementia more often. They are known to be more prone to diabetes and stroke
Lifestyle choices such as smoking and exercise	These behaviours include regular physical exercise, not smoking, drinking alcohol only in moderation (if at all), and maintaining a healthy diet and weight. The dementia risk is lowest in people who do three or more of these, not just one or two.
Type 2 diabetes and cardiovascular disease	Having cardiovascular disease or type 2 diabetes increases a person's risk of developing dementia by up to two times. These cardiovascular conditions are most strongly linked to vascular dementia. This is because vascular dementia is caused by problems with blood supply to the brain
Depression	People who have had periods of depression – whether in mid-life or later life – also seem to have increased rates of dementia. Whether depression is a risk factor that in part causes dementia is not clear, and the answer probably differs with age. There is some evidence that depression in middle age does lead to a higher dementia risk in older age.

Public Health and Health Promotion for Nurses at a Glance, First Edition. Karen Wild and Maureen McGrath.
© 2019 John Wiley & Sons Ltd. Published 2019 by John Wiley & Sons Ltd.

Introduction

The term 'dementia' describes a set of characteristics or symptoms that may include such problems as memory loss, language difficulties, and thinking and problem solving impairment (known as cognitive impairment). These changes can be a gradual process in a person, but ultimately a diagnosis is often made when the person's daily functioning becomes noticeably reduced. Alzheimer's disease is the most common cause of dementia, but not the only one. The specific symptoms that someone with dementia experiences will depend on the parts of the brain that are damaged and the disease that is causing the dementia.

- **Alzheimer's disease** is the most common cause of dementia. Proteins build up in the brain to form structures called 'plaques' and 'tangles'. Over time, chemical connections between brain cells are lost and cells begin to die. Day-to-day memory loss is often the first thing to be noticed, but other symptoms may include difficulties in finding the right words, in solving problems, in making decisions, or in perceiving things in three dimensions.
- **Vascular dementia** occurs when the oxygen supply to the brain is reduced because of narrowing or blockage of blood vessels; some brain cells become damaged or die. The symptoms can occur suddenly, following one large stroke, or they can develop over time, because of a series of small strokes. Vascular dementia affects the small blood vessels deep in the brain, and is known as subcortical vascular dementia. Many people have difficulties with problem solving or planning, thinking quickly and concentrating. They may also have short periods when they get very confused.
- **Mixed dementia** occurs when someone has more than one type of dementia, and a mixture of the symptoms of those types. It is common for someone to have both Alzheimer's disease and vascular dementia together.
- **Dementia with Lewy bodies** involves tiny abnormal structures (Lewy bodies) forming inside brain cells. They disrupt the chemistry of the brain and lead to the death of brain cells. Early symptoms can include alertness that varies over the course of the day, hallucinations and difficulties in judging distances. A person's day-to-day memory is usually affected less than in the early stages of Alzheimer's disease. Dementia with Lewy bodies is closely related to Parkinson's disease and often has some of the same symptoms, including difficulty with movement.
- **Frontotemporal dementia (including Pick's disease)** – in frontotemporal dementia the front and side parts of the brain are damaged. Clumps of abnormal proteins form inside brain cells, causing them to die. At first, changes in personality and behaviour may be the most obvious signs.
- **Rarer causes of dementia** — there are many other diseases that can lead to dementia. These are rare – together they account for only about 5% of all dementias. They tend to be more common among younger people (under age 65). These rarer causes include corticobasal degeneration, progressive supranuclear palsy, HIV infection, Niemann–Pick disease type C and Creutzfeldt–Jakob disease (CJD). Some people with Parkinson's disease or Huntington's disease develop dementia as the illness gets worse. People with Down's syndrome are also at a particular risk of developing Alzheimer's disease as they get older.

Risk factors

Several risk factors for dementia have been identified including:
- Age
- Gender
- Genetics
- Ethnicity
- Lifestyle choices such as smoking and exercise
- Hypertension
- Type 2 diabetes
- Cardiovascular disease
- Depression
- Learning disability.

Table 3.8.1 explores the risk factors in more detail.

Making every contact count

Nurses engaging in any assessment of health and wellbeing should be alerted to the early signs of dementia in order to establish the most appropriate lines of referral. Health promotion and education activities and discussions should focus on the varied risk factors identified here.

The Triangle of Care (Carers Trust, 2016) in conjunction with the Royal College of Nursing (RCN) has been developed to provide a starting point for the delivery of best care when patients have established dementia. It states that including carers in care and treatment will:

- Offer better outcomes for the person with dementia.
- Enable staff and services to ensure they have a fuller picture of the person's needs and how their dementia affects their behaviour and general wellbeing.
- Provide peace of mind for carers that the person they care for is receiving the best and appropriate treatment possible.

> *An effective Triangle of Care will only be complete if there is a willingness by the professional and carer to engage. As dementia is a progressive condition, which can affect a person's ability to make decisions for themselves and/or communicate their wishes, every effort should be made to ensure that the person with dementia is included in decision making. This requires an understanding of dementia and skill in how to support communication for people with dementia.*
>
> Carers Trust (2016)

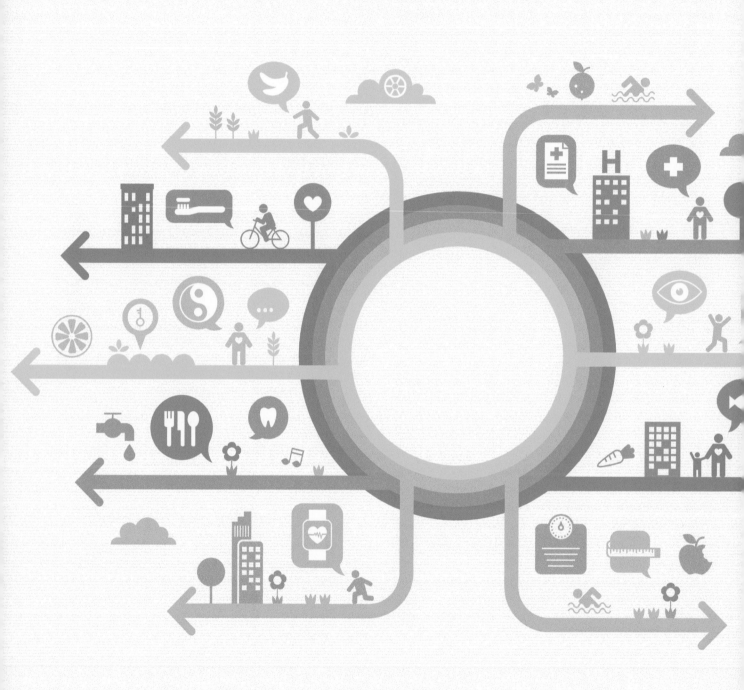

How nurses can work with individual patients to promote health

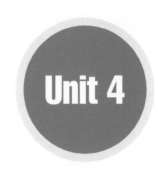

Unit 4

Chapters

Thinking points for NMC Revalidation

Having read Unit 4, reflect on your skills of communication in health promotion. Can you now identify any changes that would positively impact on your future approach with patients and clients when promoting health?

1 Why is behaviour change difficult?

Figure 4.1.1 Toolkit of behaviour change strategies. Source: Courtesy of Jane Genovese.

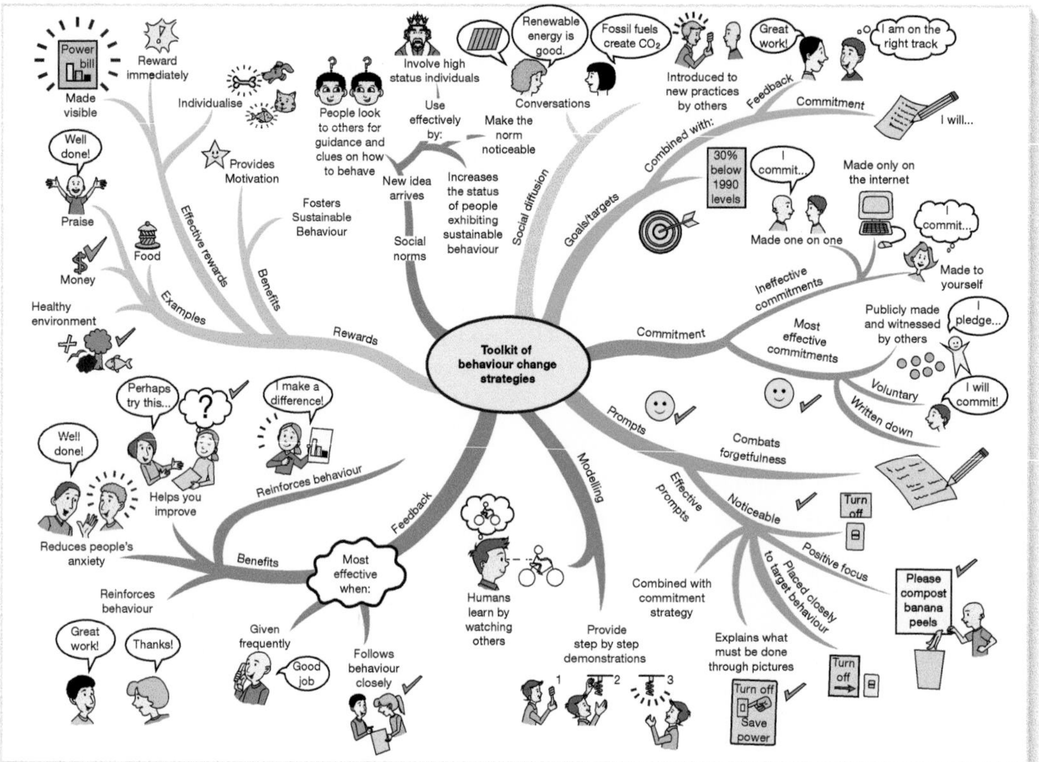

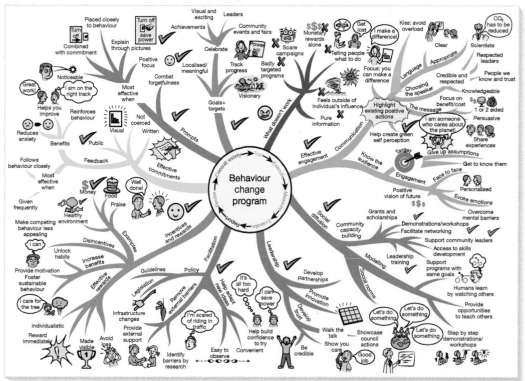

Figure 4.1.2 Elements of a behaviour change program. Source: Courtesy of Jane Genovese.

Public Health and Health Promotion for Nurses at a Glance, First Edition. Karen Wild and Maureen McGrath.

Behaviour change

For the purpose of this chapter behaviour change refers to any change in behaviour that has a positive impact on health. Parts of Unit 1 considered the nature of the major causes of mortality and morbidity in England today. Cardiovascular diseases, respiratory conditions, cancers, childhood accidents, dental caries, depression and anxiety account for the majority of ill health and premature death seen in different age groups. In addition Unit 1 also looked at the major determinants of health and considered how intrinsic factors, lifestyle and behavioural factors, social capital and wider structural factors all interact to influence behaviour and choice architecture – that is, the contexts in which people make choices and decisions about their health and health behaviour.

There has been emphasis placed by succeeding administrations on the need to support people to change behaviours that may be impacting negatively on health – for example, smoking, drinking alcohol, physical activity, eating foods high in saturated fats and sugar or high-risk sexual activity. There is also increasing recognition that people need support to learn about managing negative emotional and mental processes.

Nurses are seen to be key people in supporting individuals to change behaviour in order to improve health as detailed in documents such as Leading Change, Adding Value (NHS England, 2016); The Framework for Personalised Care and Population Health (Department of Health and Public Health England, 2014) and Making Every Contact Count (NHS Future Forum, 2012). However, despite the publication of a number of policy documents, strategies and toolkits there is little evidence that sustainable change has occurred in relation to many health behaviours. The numbers of adults and children with obesity continues to rise, the prevalence of individuals living with type 2 diabetes has grown, there has been little change in the numbers of people engaging in the recommended levels of physical activity (NHS England, 2017). Why might this be and what do nurses need to take account of when working with someone to support a change in behaviour in order to improve health?

Influences on health behaviour

As considered in Unit 1, health promotion is about a great deal more than giving out knowledge and information. People need to be able to make use of that information in the context of their own individual situation.

In this unit we will be looking at some of the established models of health behaviour and health behaviour change. These are very useful in enabling us to better understand some of the factors that influence behaviour such as perceived consequences, cues to change, attitude, subjective norms, health beliefs, motivation, self-confidence and self-efficacy. Generally all the models take account of the three ideas of causality, degree of control and perceived susceptibility and risk. It is important that nurses work to understand these different factors from the perspective of the client/patient that they are working with, and understand that every person is subject to influences that will result in different behaviours in different situations.

We are all to a large extent creatures of habit – just take a moment to think over everything you have done today. How much of it consists of things that you do in the same way on most days? These automatic responses to the day-to-day events that make our lives what they are require little conscious effort or engagement on our part and are important to our daily functioning. We respond more reflectively to those issues/problems/tasks that are outside of the everyday habits and routine of life.

It is important that nurses take account of this when working with someone to support behaviour change. The behaviour that is being addressed – for example smoking, drinking or eating a particular diet – may be an important part of the habitual daily routine that someone has or may be a key behaviour that they share with their social group. Asking someone to change may well feel equivalent to asking them to give up a key part of the person that they are or to fundamentally change the person that others perceive them to be (Kelly and Barker, 2016). This needs to be understood and discussed in terms of how this can be practically and realistically managed. Cialdini (2007) highlighted the importance of the concept of reciprocation in behaviour change — what is someone gaining in return for 'losing' an aspect of themselves?

Bouton (2014) considered that behaviour is always specific to the context in which it occurs and so behaviour change is likely to be an 'unstable and unsteady process' (p. 29).

What does this mean for nurses?

Nurses must always take account of the complex nature of behaviour change. It is important not to assume someone wants to change behaviour, and the concept of readiness to change will be considered later in this unit. It is also important that nurses engage clients/patients in a discussion about the nature of change and what might promote and hinder it. Practical suggestions about how to manage those contexts that may trigger previous behaviour patterns can be very helpful to a person undertaking some change in health behaviour.

It is important always to remember that for everyone, behaviour occurs in a social, economic and environmental context. Behaviour change therefore has the potential to be overwhelmingly complex. Figures 4.1.1 and 4.1.2 illustrate this complexity diagrammatically. In order to make change realistic and to have the potential to be sustainable nurses should understand the contexts that are relevant for individual patients and clients. They should therefore 'Make Every Contact Count' (NHS Future Forum, 2012) through taking every opportunity to **learn** about the contexts within which clients/patients live.

2 Models of health behaviour

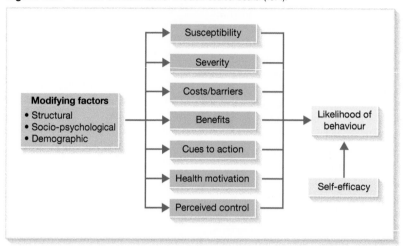

Figure 4.2.1 Becker's health belief model. Source: Becker (1974).

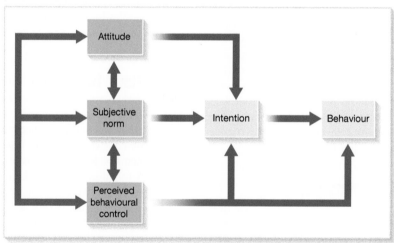

Figure 4.2.2 Theory of planned behaviour model. Source: Ajzen (1991). Reproduced with permission of Elsevier.

Box 4.2.1 Tones' Health Action Model. Source: Data from Tones (1987) in Tones and Green (2010).

Takes account of:
- **Beliefs**
- **Motivation**
- **Normative influences**
- **Self**

Proposes that they all interact to determine likelihood of **intention**.

Whether **intention** translates into **action** depends on a number of enabling or limiting factors including knowledge, skills (+ self-efficacy) and the environment.

Public Health and Health Promotion for Nurses at a Glance, First Edition. Karen Wild and Maureen McGrath.
© 2019 John Wiley & Sons Ltd. Published 2019 by John Wiley & Sons Ltd.

Relevance of the models to nurses

Most people have 'go to' behaviours that will occur or be increased when stressed, distressed or anxious. These are many and varied and include eating, drinking alcohol, drinking coffee, smoking, sex, shopping, electronic gaming or box set binges. Just take a moment to identify your own 'go to' behaviour. As stated in Chapter 1 of this unit, these behaviours can become habitual. It is thought by some that certain behaviours impact on the brain's motivation and reward system in the same way that some substances do and so can be become 'addictive' behaviours. This may have implications for how people should best be supported to make changes, and nurses need to be aware of this view. However, they can use communication skills and practical advice to help people appropriately and opportunistically. It should also be remembered that nurses may be promoting the uptake of a health behaviour for some people, such as starting a medication regime.

Figures 4.2.1 and 4.2.2 and Box 4.2.1 illustrate the models of health behaviour that are most commonly reflected in the literature on health behaviours and in policy/Cabinet Office documents (The Behavioural Insights Team, 2016; NICE, 2014). The literature also indicates the limitations of the models, and they should be considered as one of many useful tools available to nurses in their practice. Chapter 1 identified that the factors/theories informing the models of health behaviour can largely be summarised under three categories: causality, degree of control and perceived susceptibility and risk.

Causality

Dave is 55 years old and works in retail. In conversation with a nurse he talks about the reasons for his drinking behaviour. He was raised in a home in which alcohol was a part of everyday life – both parents drank regularly, alcohol was always bought as part of any trip to the shop, all social occasions involved alcohol, and his current partner and friends are all regular drinkers. For Dave drinking alcohol is the 'norm'. He perceives drinking alcohol to be part of who he is and a part of how others see him. He enjoys this behaviour. The nurse might want to explore this further by asking if Dave (or his friends/family) has suffered any negative consequences from drink being such a big part of his/their lives.

'Has anything ever happened as a result of drinking that you or someone you know has regretted?'

Here the nurse is starting to explore the perception of cost of this behaviour as well as potential cues to action.

Degree of control

The health visitor is in conversation with Rachel, aged 19, following the birth of her baby Jayden. Rachel is severely obese (BMI 35) and says she is desperate to lose weight but says that she has been on diets all of her life without success. She does not want to be Jayden's 'fat mum' and does not want him to be overweight. Rachel is expressing a 'cue for action' that she has identified and is also saying that she does not perceive herself as having very much control over losing her weight. The health visitor picks up that Rachel is motivated to lose weight in that she seems to have made a choice that she wants to lose weight for particular reasons at this time. However, she does not seem to have the confidence to change and address potential barriers to change (self-efficacy). The health visitor would want to clarify Rachel's previous experiences of weight loss:

'When you say you have been on diets all your life – does that mean from being a young child?'

'What different diets have you tried and what happened?'

'What weight would you aim to be?'

In this way the health visitor may get insight into some of the reasons for Rachel's obesity and the factors that stop her losing weight, and might ask further questions about these. The health visitor would aim to develop Rachel's belief in her ability to lose weight (her self-efficacy). This may come about through encouragement from people in a similar position to herself at a weight loss group – one of the established commercial groups or one organised by health visitors for women with young babies.

Perceived susceptibility and risk

Jordan is 13 years old and was diagnosed with epilepsy when he was 7 years old following a series of tonic-clonic seizures. Jordan's epilepsy was well controlled with antiepileptic medication and at age 10 years Jordan was taken off his medication and had not experienced any seizures until a month ago. He has had three tonic-clonic seizures in the last month, two of these have occurred at school. Jordan demonstrates maturity and the capacity to understand his condition and treatment. He tells you that he does not wish to start antiepileptic medication again as it took some time to find the medication that suited him best last time. Also he is doing well academically and is also involved in a number of sports. He has read on the internet about the side effects of antiepileptic drugs and feels he did suffer from some of these previously. He feels the recent seizures were due to his getting overtired and that if he avoids this he will be OK. The nurse practitioner might want to ask Jordan questions (with his parents' permission) in order to explore the risk of future seizures and Jordan's susceptibility to harm as a result of these.

'Can you tell me more about the recent seizures – how you felt before and after them, and how long they lasted?'

'What would it mean for your school sports activities if the seizures continue?'

'What would make you feel more comfortable about starting medication again?'

'Do you know anyone who is managing their epilepsy with medication at present?'

Models and theories of behaviour change

3

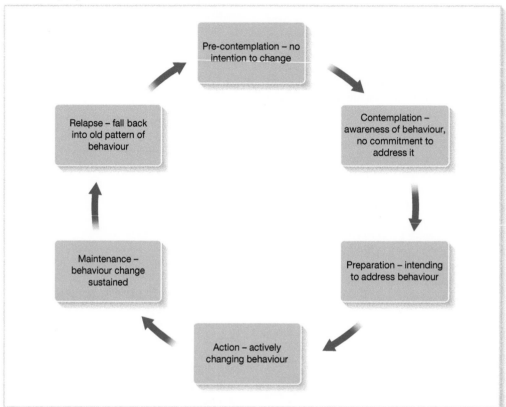

Figure 4.3.1 Transtheoretical model of behaviour change/cycles of change model. Source: Data from Prochaska and Diclimente (1984).

- Pre-contemplation – no intention to change
- Contemplation – awareness of behaviour, no commitment to address it
- Preparation – intending to address behaviour
- Action – actively changing behaviour
- Maintenance – behaviour change sustained
- Relapse – fall back into old pattern of behaviour

Box 4.3.1 Nudge theory of behaviour change. Source: Data from Thaler and Sunstein (2009).

- Make the **DEFAULT** option the healthier option.
- Take account of influence of:
  - REPRESENTATIVENESS
  - AVAILABILITY
  - ANCHORING

Box 4.3.2 Influence and persuasion in behaviour change. Source: Data from Cialdini (2007).

Key factors to consider when supporting a person with a behaviour change:

- Reciprocation
- Commitment and consistency
- Social proof
- Liking
- Authority
- Scarcity

Public Health and Health Promotion for Nurses at a Glance, First Edition. Karen Wild and Maureen McGrath.
© 2019 John Wiley & Sons Ltd. Published 2019 by John Wiley & Sons Ltd.

How nurses can use the models and theories

In Chapter 2 of this unit the focus was on trying to understand health behaviour from the perspective of the patient or client. What should be avoided at all costs is simply pointing out what is wrong or 'bad' about a behaviour or simply stating what a person **should** do. Most people are already aware of these facts, and the real issue is why change is so difficult despite that knowledge. In this chapter we will look at some issues that nurses might want to explore with someone who has demonstrated that they are ready to make a change in some aspect of their health behaviour.

Nudge theory of behaviour change

This theory (Box 4.3.1) promotes the idea of making small realistic changes to influence health behaviour for the better, rather than attempting a complete behaviour change at a point in time. If someone is ready to make changes to increase their levels of physical activity, then deciding to walk 15 minutes every day might be a more sustainable change than attending three classes a week at the local gym. Walking 15 minutes daily might be achieved through getting off public transport at a stop before the one normally used, using stairs rather than lifts, walking to local shops rather than driving, walking the dog or walking the children to school. These activities have no financial cost, require no expensive clothing and will be less time consuming than a trip to the gym. Someone may wish to develop goals that are related to regular sport and activity, but starting off with realistic achievable changes is likely to result in commitment and in people feeling good about the change that they have been able to make and sustain. This theory has influenced the government-funded Change4Life campaign (Public Health England, 2018).

The theory suggests a number of influences that need to be taken account of when promoting health improvement. People are influenced by what they see to be **representative patterns of health**. Suppose a respiratory specialist nurse is encouraging a patient with chronic obstructive pulmonary disease to have the 'flu' (influenza) vaccine. The patient might make a decision based on the fact that he does not know anyone who has had 'flu' apart from those who have had the vaccine and then been ill, The influenza vaccine is an inactivated vaccine and cannot 'cause' flu but can often cause flu-like symptoms, particularly if someone has a virus for a minor illness but is presymptomatic at the time of the 'flu' injection. The nurse would need to take time to explain the difference between this and the very serious symptoms that influenza may cause.

Another influence on people's understanding of their health and their motivation to change is what the theory refers to as **availability** – by which is meant someone's view or perception of what an illness or a health behaviour is. If someone perceives that depression is an illness that causes people to stay in bed all day, weeping and unable to function, they may not recognise the link between their own mental health and symptoms such as lethargy, difficulties in socialising or sleep problems. Another person may be confident that they do not have a problem with their use of alcohol because they never drink before 6 pm. It is important that nurses explore what a person understands by the medical terms and labels used for illness and for health behaviours in order to support someone to make sustainable changes.

Another important influence is **anchoring** – people base their ideas about risks associated with health behaviours on what they see in their immediate social group. Someone may tell the nurse that everyone in their family is overweight/obese and they are all healthy and have lived into their 80s. This view will have an impact on a person's motivation and self-efficacy, both of which are necessary to effect and sustain change. The nurse would just accept this information and discuss again with the patient why **they** have decided to make a change and what that will mean to **them**, as well as reminding them of previous discussions about the advantages of being a healthy weight.

Cialdini's work on behaviour change

An important element of Cialdini's (2007) work is the idea of **reciprocation** (Box 4.3.2). As indicated in earlier chapters, some changes in health behaviour may significantly impact on the sense of individual personhood as perceived by self and others. It is very important that nurses understand this and work with people to identify clearly what the tangible gains are for any individual in making a change. These need to be revisited regularly as change is sustained. Other important elements in change are **social proof**, the idea that people are more likely to be persuaded to change if others in the same social group or others seen to be similar to themselves change. This might help explain the success of quit smoking support groups or weight loss groups. Cialdini (2007) says that people who make a public **commitment** to change are likely to be more successful. Also, if people can be made aware of the limitations (**scarcity**) that a behaviour is causing for them then this may help – for example using spirometry to indicate reduced lung capacity in a person who smokes regularly. Nurses should also take account of the elements of **liking** and **authority**. People engaging with complex change respond best when supported by people with whom they develop a working relationship and who are knowledgeable and authoritative regarding the area of change concerned.

Transtheoretical model of behaviour change

This model (Figure 4.3.1) is commonly used in nursing texts and in practice. It will be considered in more depth in the chapters looking at skills to support behaviour change in this unit (Chapters 6–9). It stresses the idea that change takes time and can involve 'relapses' to the original behaviour that is being changed; different support skills can be used for support at different stages.

4 Readiness to change

Figure 4.4.1 COM-B (Capability, Opportunity, Motivation – Behaviour) readiness to change conditions.
Source: Adapted from Michie *et al.*, (2011).

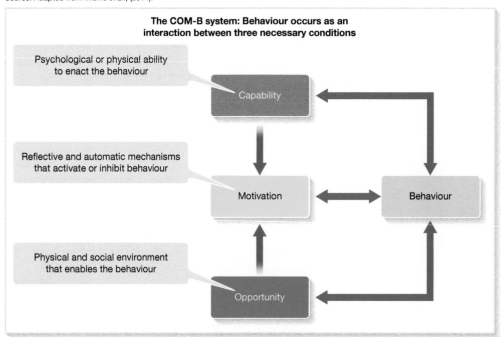

Figure 4.4.2 Factors that influence readiness to change (NICE, 2007; Dixon, 2008).

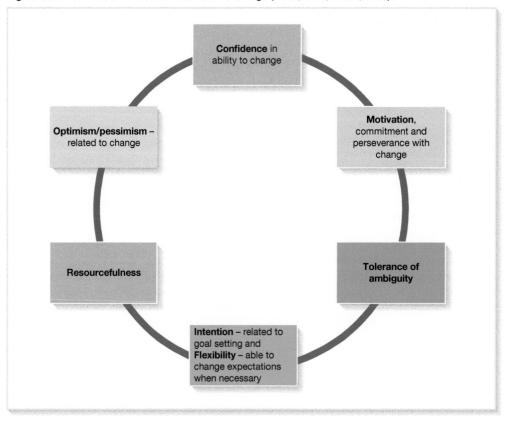

Public Health and Health Promotion for Nurses at a Glance, First Edition. Karen Wild and Maureen McGrath.
© 2019 John Wiley & Sons Ltd. Published 2019 by John Wiley & Sons Ltd.

What is readiness to change?

Readiness to change is a concept referred to regularly in clinical areas and is often used to consider the success or failure of an episode of care (Dalton and Gottlieb, 2003). We might speak of someone being

- 'ready for discharge'
- 'not ready to fully accept diagnosis'
- 'not ready to engage with care plan/proposed intervention'
- 'ready to engage in behaviour change'.

Any patient's readiness to engage with a change in behaviour or circumstances is always context driven and always related to an outcome (some examples are, becoming independent, feeling well, able to work again). Readiness should be considered as both a state and a process. The process of becoming ready is influenced by a large number of factors, both internal and external to the individual (Figures 4.4.1 and 4.4.2) and different factors will be more significant for people at different stages in the process of becoming ready to make a change. Nurses working with people who are making a change (e.g. in lifestyle behaviour, in management of medication, in developing self-awareness or social skills) need to be continually assessing a person's motivation to change, their perceived capability and confidence and any opportunities that arise that promote or threaten change (Figure 4.4.1). They also need to be encouraging a person to recognise factors intrinsic to them that will enable them to sustain a change and sharing techniques that might promote development of some of these factors (Figure 4.4.2).

The nurse's role in assessing clients' readiness

Dalton and Gottlieb (2003) in their paper on the concept of readiness to change suggest a number of important aspects of the role of the nurse in supporting a person in changing a health behaviour.

Work collaboratively

The nurse should work as an equal partner in the endeavour of change and not as 'the expert' dispensing advice. The views and perspectives of the patient making the change should always be central and the nurse should work to affirm and encourage self-efficacy, continually acknowledging the awareness and effort of the patient. In this way the nurse would be promoting the patient's capability to make changes (Figure 4.4.1), and this may then impact positively on motivation to change and on the actual behaviour change. Positive behaviour change in turn may then positively impact on capability, motivation and opportunity. For example, genuinely offering positive regard ('well done – that is a real difference to the last time we met'; 'you look well, how do you feel?') to someone who has started to improve physical activity levels by walking for 10 minutes every day may reinforce their belief that they **can** make changes, may strengthen their determination to continue to walk every day and may encourage them to actively create opportunities to walk for 10 minutes (or more!) every day next week. This joint acknowledgement of success will also impact on the factors of confidence, optimism and adventurousness (Figure 4.4.2).

Discern when support starts to feel like pressure

Within any therapeutic relationship there exists the danger that the patient may want to 'please' the nurse in the sense of continuing to achieve agreed goals of change. It is important that the nurse is sensitive to this and continually places the ownership of agreed goals with the patient and conveys that support is offered for what the patient agrees they can do and not for what the nurse expects them to do. Starting conversations by asking, 'So, how are you this week?' rather than, 'So, how have you done with the goals we set last time?' is one way of conveying this approach. Sometimes people may reach a stage where they cannot make more change at the present time, and this also needs to be acknowledged through exploration of the situation and empathy. Failure to work in this way can negatively impact on motivation (Figure 4.4.1) and on flexibility, resourcefulness, resilience and passion (Figure 4.4.2). It is important that the pace of change is dictated by the patient.

Explore ambivalence

Change is difficult, as indicated in earlier chapters, and most people will be able to hold more than one view of any change they are attempting. For example, someone may say, 'I know that I feel better for walking every day but it is just too hard to find time to do it'. It is important to explore in depth what is meant by 'feel better' and how important that is to someone and those around them and also to discuss what is meant by 'finding time'. Is this every day or just some days? What other things are taking priority? Can these be managed differently? Ambivalence may impact on motivation and on the creating of opportunities to carry out behaviour change (Figure 4.4.1) and on tolerance of ambiguity (Figure 4.4.2).

Focus on the manageable

Change can often feel overwhelming. Someone may have made great progress towards a goal but this may be impacted by the simple fact that 'life happens' to everyone. The patient who is improving their physical activity may suddenly have to provide care for an older relative. Their energy levels and time availability may mean they cannot walk everyday. It is important then to consider what **can** they do. They may only be able to walk once or twice a week. This still helps them to feel better but is realistic in the current circumstances. If a change feels unmanageable this may impact on capability and motivation (Figure 4.4.1) and on passion, resourcefulness and optimism (Figure 4.4.2).

Develop awareness of negativity

When the sustainability of change is hard people will focus on the negative impact of behaviour change for them. The nurse should explore this by just asking questions that make someone aware of it. For example, 'Are there any positives that result from this change?' 'How important are they compared with the negatives you are recognising?' Unchallenged negativity will impact on capability, motivation and opportunity for change (Figure 4.4.1) and on confidence and optimism (Figure 4.4.2).

5 Self-efficacy and resilience

Figure 4.5.1 Self-efficacy. Source: Data from Bandura (1997).

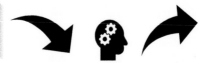

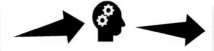

Influences		Outcomes
Performance Outcomes (Mastery) – related to previous successes or failures in changing behaviour		**Confidence** – in ability to make a change
Vicarious Experiences – observation of the successes (or failures) of others – particularly influential people		**Effort and Perseverance** – someone is willing to make to effect a change
Verbal Persuasion – encouragement (or discouragement) offered by others, particularly influential people		**Perception** – someone has of their ability to make a change
Physiological Feedback – the state of a person's physical or mental wellbeing		**Self-assurance and Self-reliance** – regarding the resources available to someone to help them make a change

Table 4.5.1 Some resilience factors. Source: Adapted from Pemberton (2015); and Reivich and Shatte (2003).

Factor	What does this mean?
Self-belief and self-efficacy	Awareness of personal strengths and weaknesses. Ability to use this awareness to achieve goals/outcomes
Flexibility	Able to view situations and circumstances from a number of perspectives
Solution finding	Acting on problems rather than ignoring them; drawing on variety of resources to problem solve
Receiving support	Connecting with others. Able to ask for support, confide in others. Able to delegate
Emotional awareness and control	Able to acknowledge emotions, label them and manage them appropriately
Realistic positivity	Perceiving self and situation as positively as possible within any particular context
Learning to be comfortable with uncertainty	Accepting that it is not possible to have control and certainty regarding every aspect of our lives

Public Health and Health Promotion for Nurses at a Glance, First Edition. Karen Wild and Maureen McGrath.
© 2019 John Wiley & Sons Ltd. Published 2019 by John Wiley & Sons Ltd.

Self-efficacy, resilience and behaviour change

Self-efficacy

There is evidence to show that interventions that promote self-efficacy can be successful in sustaining a positive health behaviour (Schwarzer and Warner, 2013). Self-efficacy is also an important component of both the models that attempt to explain health behaviours and the models of behaviour change (see Chapters 2 and 3 of this unit, and Figure 4.5.1). Self-efficacy reflects an optimism that novel or difficult tasks can be completed and that desired outcomes can be achieved. It reflects a confidence in the ability to deal with life's challenges. It might be thought of as a way of being (in relation to particular behavioural outcomes) that reflects a belief in being able to control and shape one's personal future and attain desired outcomes due to one's own actions and decisions (Bandura, 1997). Perceived behavioural control and self-efficacy are both concepts that relate to an individual's belief in being able to attain certain behavioural outcomes. Perceived behavioural control might refer more to the ease or difficulty of attaining the outcomes whereas self-efficacy relates to the belief that the outcomes **can** be attained. A person can demonstrate self-efficacy in some situations and not in others.

Resilience

Resilience is the ability to cope adaptively with traumatic stressors and is seen as comprising other personal resources such as self-esteem, self-efficacy, optimism, coping strategies and social relations (Table 4.5.1) (Antonovsky, 1987; Schwarzer and Warner, 2013). A person's level of resilience reflects levels of physiological and psychological functioning, which may only be evident in the presence of particular stressors. People may demonstrate resilience to some stressors and not others, and it is important to see resilience as something that can evolve and develop. Most research on resilience indicates that early childhood experiences with key care givers are central to an individual's levels of resilience (Hill et al., 2007). Given the nature of the personal resources that contribute to levels of resilience (Table 4.5.1) there would be potential to work with someone to develop these resources in relation to a specific health behaviour that was being developed or maintained and self-efficacy is one of these.

Interventions to support the development of self-efficacy in relation to a health behaviour

Bandura (1997) identified four major influences on the generation of self-efficacy (Figure 4.5.1).

1. Mastery experience (performance outcomes)

This relates to an individual's previous experiences in relation to a health behaviour: previous success fosters self-efficacy whereas previous failure undermines self-efficacy. Someone may tell a nurse that they have 'given up' smoking lots of times previously only to start again and that they have concluded that they will never be able to quit smoking for good. The nurse can listen and express empathy with this view, discussing how difficult change is and how most people 'quit' several times before quitting smoking for good. It would be important to look at what the reasons were for quitting previously and what had helped them be successful for a time. It would also be important to ask about the reasons for starting to smoke again. This might enable a plan to be made that would facilitate quitting and develop strategies to minimise the risk of starting again. Continued focus on any success is important in encouraging sustained success

2. Vicarious experience

Seeing other people succeed in making a behaviour change can be important in providing exposure to strategies and techniques that might be helpful in achieving set goals and in overcoming obstacles to those goals. This may explain why support groups are important in encouraging and sustaining change for some people; examples are weight loss groups for adults and MEND/SHINE weight loss programmes for children and their families; 'stop smoking' groups; Alcoholics Anonymous; and mental health support groups. Attendance at a support group may be an important goal for the individual and their nurse to agree.

3. Verbal persuasion/social persuasion

If a person receives consistent encouragement from someone who genuinely expresses faith in their ability to change and capability to achieve goals their self-efficacy is promoted. This is an important role for the nurse who is supporting someone to sustain a change. So a nurse may say something like, 'Well, I know you are disappointed not to have lost as much weight as you have been doing, but it is important to think about how much you have lost overall and not to expect that you will lose the same amount every week. Think about how much better you are feeling and how much nearer your goal you are.' It might also be important to help someone develop strategies to counter sources of discouragement.

4. Perceptions of somatic/affective states (physiological feedback)

A person's physical and emotional state will impact on how ready they are to make a behavioural change. If someone is physically unwell or if their emotional wellbeing is impacted by loss, grief or anxiety, it may not be an appropriate time to embark on behaviour change as the change itself is likely to require reserves of both physical and emotional energy. Someone recovering from physical or mental ill health may, however, be in an ideal position to start to make some changes as their motivation and determination may be high – particularly if they are focusing on changing a behaviour that contributed to their illness. It is important that nurses have conversations with people about these issues. It is also important to explore with people the impact that their current behaviour has on them – both physically and also on how they feel, their moods and attitudes. Someone may say that the behaviour that they are thinking of changing actually makes them feel better, at least in the short term. It would therefore be important to identify what they would be gaining by changing this behaviour, both in the short and long term, and to develop clear goals related to this. As these goals are achieved self-efficacy is promoted.

6 Skills to support behaviour change

Figure 4.6.1 Six characteristics of brief intervention (BI) – FRAMES.

- **Feedback**: about personal risk or impairment
- **Responsibility**: an emphasis on personal responsibility for change
- **Advice**: to manage behaviour differently
- **Menu**: of alternative options for change and goal setting
- **Empathic interviewing**: 'being with' the person where they are
- **Self-efficacy**: promoted by an interviewing style that enhances belief in the ability to change

↓

Example: 'I know I am going to get all these medicines mixed up.'

- **Feedback**: 'What do you know about your medicines?' 'What do you think will happen if you do get the medicines mixed up?' 'How does that idea make you feel?'
- **Responsibility**: 'What things can you do to be able to manage your medicines safely?' 'What will help you do this?'
- **Advice**: 'Some patients arrange with their pharmacist to organise their medication either with charts or with dosage boxes?' 'Who could help you with this?'
- **Menu**: 'So there seems to be some options to help you with this. We can speak with the pharmacist here before your discharge. Your son could speak to your local pharmacist about organising medication when you are home. Your son will help you to get used to your medication following discharge.' 'Is there other help you might need to manage this?'
- **Empathic interviewing**: 'It can be really overwhelming to be faced with managing new medicines in order to stay well, most people would find it confusing initially. The important thing is to know who you can contact for help particularly in the early days after discharge.' 'Do you feel any clearer about who could help you?'
- **Self-efficacy**: 'You have done so well since coming on to the unit. You have been determined to be independent and get home again as soon as possible. I feel sure that you will be more confident about your medicines before discharge and we will start to enable you to manage them from hereon.'

Public Health and Health Promotion for Nurses at a Glance, First Edition. Karen Wild and Maureen McGrath.

Guidance, not advice; listening, not telling

Nurses in busy clinical situations have a professional responsibility to spend time wisely and effectively and in ways that best help the patient/client they are supporting. Advice/instruction/direction about health behaviour is very often ineffective and is likely to promote resistance if done in isolation. A guiding style of engagement that encourages the patient to identify what feels right for them and to determine why and how they might make changes will be more effective for many people (Rollnick et al., 2010). However, the issue facing many nurses is the time constraint on all aspects of their work. It is important that nurses develop skills and tools that help them to engage in realistic 'change talk' with people over a relatively short period of time. All nurses can develop skills to engage in the techniques of brief interventions and motivational interviewing.

Brief intervention (BI)

This technique can help nurses effectively respond to a comment that a person makes to them, such as:

- 'I know I am going to get all these medicines mixed up.'
- 'I cannot see me being able to lose weight to help my diabetes.'
- 'I really want to try and stop smoking now.'

Brief interventions typically take between 5 and 15 minutes and involve opportunistic assessment (of commitment to change), discussion, negotiation, encouragement and advice. They are structured conversations in which the nurse may guide the direction of the conversation while the patient/client retains responsibility for any proposed change. The intervention uses the skills of motivational interviewing (Miller and Rollnick, 2002; National Institute for Health and Care Excellence, 2006; World Health Organization, 2010; National Obesity Observatory, 2011). Miller and Sanchez (1994) identified six characteristics that should be evident in all brief interventions (Figure 4.6.1), and the 5As model lists key strategies for completing a BI (World Health Organization, 2014). These are:

- Ask
- Assess
- Advise
- Assist
- Arrange follow-up.

Motivational interviewing

The technique of motivational interviewing enables nurses to work in collaboration with people emphasising their autonomy over decision making and eliciting their motivation for change (Rollnick et al., 2010). The aim if working in this way is to encourage a rapid engagement to focus on realistic changes that can make a difference for the individual concerned. The nurse retains control over the direction and structure of the consultation in order to manage the constraints of time and other clinical responsibilities, but the patient always retains the responsibility for change. There are some key principles and key skills that should be characteristic of all motivational interviewing, helpfully these are often expressed as acronyms.

RULE (Rollnick et al., 2008; Rosengren, 2009)

The key principles are that the nurse should:

R – resist the righting reflex. The nurse should avoid the inclination to 'fix' or to put right the person's behaviour. The nurse is not directing but guiding; not instilling change but helping elicit the motivation to change.

U – understand and explore the patient's own motivations. What do they gain from their current behaviour? What are the positives and negatives associated with it? What would it mean to change this behaviour? What would be the consequences of doing this? What would they gain? What would they lose through a change? What is most important to them at present?

L – listen with empathy. The patient should do most of the talking in the interview. The nurse should not be challenging or arguing with things the patient says. The nurse's responses should demonstrate understanding and show that active listening is taking place.

'It is interesting to hear you say how worried you are about your children seeing you smoke and yet you say you cannot manage more than a couple of hours without a cigarette. What difficulties does that cause for you?'

'Change is always very difficult and is rarely a once and for all event, it is more of a process and can be affected by a number of things.'

E – empower the patient. The nurse should encourage hope, optimism and self-efficacy (see Chapter 5 of this unit).

OARS (Miller and Rollnick, 2002)

The key skills that the nurse should use are:

O – open-ended questioning. These questions encourage a considered and thoughtful response that will be more helpful than a yes/no answer.

A – affirmations. To affirm achievements, personal strengths or abilities the nurse has to actively and carefully listen to the patient.

'You have a lot of insight into the reasons why you drink more in particular social situations.'

'It may feel like a very small change but it is such an important first step.'

'It is good to see you again, how are you?'

R – reflective listening. This skill is really important in increasing a patient's self-awareness. The nurse may just reflect the patient's own words back to them: 'You stopped your diet for a couple of days last week because work was so busy.' The patient's feelings may be reflected back to them: 'You felt angry because you feel you are taken for granted at work' or 'You sound upset when you speak about the impact on your husband.'

S – summarising. The nurse should briefly summarise the conversation/discussion to make sure that both parties agree on what has been discussed, and where appropriate this summary will include agreed realistic and achievable goals to move towards sustainable behaviour change. See if you can identify any of these skills in Figure 4.6.1.

7 Skills supporting behaviour change. Example 1: Jenna

Figure 4.7.1 Becker's Health Belief model.

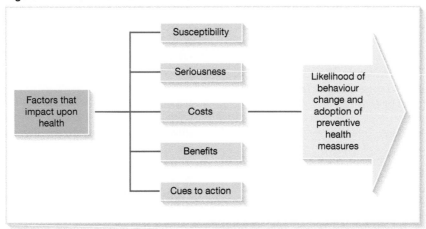

Table 4.7.1 Concepts, definition and application of Becker's model.

Concept	Definition	Application
Perceived susceptibility	One's opinion of chances of getting a condition	Define population(s) at risk, risk levels; personalise risk based on a person's features or behavior; heighten perceived susceptibility if too low.
Perceived severity	One's opinion of how serious a condition and its consequences are	Specify consequences of the risk and the condition.
Perceived benefits	One's belief in the efficacy of the advised action to reduce risk or seriousness of impact	Define action to take; how, where, when; clarify the positive effects to be expected.
Perceived barriers	One's opinion of the tangible and psychological costs of the advised action	Identify and reduce barriers through reassurance, incentives, assistance.
Cues to action	Strategies to activate "readiness"	Provide how-to information, promote awareness, reminders.
Self-efficacy	Confidence in one's ability to take action	Provide training, guidance in performing action.

Case study.

Jenna, aged 49, is really anxious about attending for cervical screening. For some time she has been experiencing discomfort during intercourse, feeling sore, and not enjoying sex with her partner any longer.

At the screening session, the practice nurse, Sue, notices Jenna's anxiety, picking up on her body language, which is tense and edgy.

- **Sue:** 'You just seem a little bit anxious, are you feeling OK about what we are about to do?'
- **Jenna:** 'I'm absolutely dreading this, its been on my mind for days.' Jenna looks away and starts to be tearful.
- **Sue:** 'I'm really sorry that you've felt like that, do want to tell me why you have been feeling so worried about it?'
- **Jenna:** 'I just feel really embarrassed talking to somebody about this, a bit silly really at my age.'
- **Sue:** 'That's OK. I understand it can be like that; a lot of women feel the same; is there anything that I can help you with?

Public Health and Health Promotion for Nurses at a Glance, First Edition. Karen Wild and Maureen McGrath.
© 2019 John Wiley & Sons Ltd. Published 2019 by John Wiley & Sons Ltd.

77

Chapter 7 Skills supporting behaviour change. Example 1: Jenna

Becker's Health Belief model (Becker, 1974) is an adaptive tool that can be used by nurses to support people in relation to their health behaviours. As such it is identified as a behavioural model of health with its roots firmly planted in social psychology. It was initially formulated by Rosenstock (1966), and was developed further by Becker in the next couple of decades (Figure 4.7.1).

Behavioural models of health, like Becker's, focus on aspects of the determinants of health (identified in Unit 1, Chapter 3), in particular health beliefs that individuals or groups may have towards certain aspects of lifestyle behaviours such as:

* The types of diet and the levels of exercise people may have.
* Smoking behaviour.
* Response to stresses in life.
* Sexual health behaviour.

Becker's model is based on the understanding that a person will take positive steps towards their health if:

1 They feel that a negative health issue can be prevented.
2 They have a perception that by acting on their health there will be a positive outcome.
3 They perceive that they can successfully take advice and manage their health.

Becker's Health Belief model

This model focuses on a set of core health beliefs that are felt to strongly influence health behaviour. There are five core beliefs:

* Susceptibility to illness
* Seriousness of any consequences of behaviour
* Cost to the individual
* Benefits to the individual
* Cues to action.

Behavioural approaches have a focus on the link between health and behaviour. Health promotion using behavioural approaches is likely to include the giving of information by the nurse, and the development of methods to use that information in order to promote health in everyday life situations.

Application of the model: case study

In the case study (see Case study) Jenna is presenting for routine cervical screening. What is evident to the practice nurse, Sue, is Jenna's behaviour, and Sue clearly wants to engage with Jenna to understand that behaviour.

What are the different issues that the scenario in the Case study raises from the point of view of:

* Sue the practice nurse?
* Jenna the patient?

From Sue's point of view, it is important that Jenna has the cervical screen that she has attended for. However, what Sue picks up on when engaging with Jenna is the presence of other potential health issues.

Health Belief and cervical screening

* **Susceptibility to illness:** as a 49-year-old woman who has been sexually active, Jenna understands her risk of developing cervical cancer.
* **Seriousness of any consequences of behaviour:** Jenna knows that cervical cancer is a serious life-threatening disease that can be detected at an early stage through screening. She is aware that missing the screening opportunity could have serious health consequences.
* **Cost to the individual:** Jenna is really anxious about the discomfort that she may experience as part of this procedure
* **Benefits to the individual:** Having a negative result will give her peace of mind and reassure her about some aspects of her sexual wellbeing, e.g. possible infection.
* **Cues to action:** Jenna has been invited to attend, and despite her anxieties around her sexual health, has attended.

During the conversation with Jenna, Sue is able to pick up on the problems that Jenna is experiencing during sexual intercourse. Sue's style and approach are reflective of the key skills that are required in motivational interviewing and part of what Sue will be doing is assessing Jenna's readiness to look at this issue further and to explore the possible options available to her.

Health Belief and Jenna's sexual health

* **Susceptibility to illness:** Jenna may be worried that her symptoms are a result of some physical abnormality or disease.
* **Seriousness of any consequences of behaviour:** Jenna may be really worried that if this carries on, she will no longer feel able to engage in intercourse with her partner, and that this may have serious consequences for her relationship.
* **Cost to the individual:** her immediate feelings may be in terms of the dread, fear and anxiety. She may also worry that investigation of a potential physical problem might mean time out from work and its impact on friends and family.
* **Benefits to the individual:** contextualising and naming the problem for Jenna helps her to understand and come to terms with what is a common and treatable issue.
* **Cues to action:** the deterioration of her sexual enjoyment and the real worry that something may be seriously wrong.

The model and its application (Table 4.7.1) provide the nurse with a structure with which to understand the issue from Jenna's perspective, to work with Jenna to support her through the cervical screen and to promote her sexual health.

8 Skills supporting behaviour change. Example 2: Rachel

Box 4.8.1 Exploring Rachel's readiness to change.

HV: 'It can be really discouraging when you lose weight and then gain it again. How much weight would you like to lose. Do you have a goal?'
Rachel: 'Well I'd like to be a size 10 rather than a size 22 (laughs). But I would be happy to lose a couple of stone and keep it off.'

Here the HV is expressing empathy with Rachel and affirming the difficulties people have in sustaining weight loss. Identifying a specific goal to aim for is an important aspect of Rachel taking control of the situation and being ready to change

Box 4.8.3 How proposed plan addresses some of factors supporting behaviour change.

The plan to look at arranging a prescription referral to a weight loss class and an exercise programme locally may support the following:
- **Reciprocation:** Rachel may feel that engaging in this plan will help enable her become the mum she wants to be and also feel better about herself
- **Social proof:** Being with other people who are in some way similar to herself, with similar goals, who '*speak her language*' in relation to weight loss may encourage her
- **Commitment:** Attendance at the classes is a public commitment about what Rachel wants to achieve and she may develop a commitment to the group of people she meets, which may help sustain changes
- **Scarcity:** Rachel has talked about her weight 'limiting' her in different ways and wanting this to be different. This plan may be a way of reducing those limitations

Box 4.8.2 Reason's for Rachel's behaviour.

HV: 'Does trying to lose 2 stones sound achievable and realistic to you?'
Rachel: 'Yes I think so. I mean I've lost a lot more than that in the past – I got down to twelve-and-a-half stones once, but I put it all back on again. All of us in our family are overweight, my mum, my sister, my sister's kids – its just how we are and a lot of the time I accept it but some things do upset me. I've not always felt OK about doing things with my friends – like going to festivals, or going shopping. I do also remember kids at school calling us names, and I know it is not healthy to be this weight. It's not just about wanting to be skinny, I want to be proud of myself and I want Jayden to be proud of me.'
HV: 'So, what diets have you tried in the past?'
Rachel: 'You name it and I've tried it – low carb, low fat, fasting diets, meal replacement diets – but I've never been able to stick at them for long. It is just really hard to keep it up and I end up giving myself a treat and that's it I've blown it and am back to snacking all the time and eating what I really love – fry-ups, pastries, pies, chips. I kid myself that the diets are expensive – but I spend so much money on rubbish. My partner is slim and he cycles everywhere – so he can eat what he wants.'
HV: 'I think lots of people could identify with what you say – it is really tough trying to make any long-term change to our behaviour. It is clear though that you feel determined to make some changes – not just for you but for Jayden also.'

The HV is gaining some insight into Rachel's behaviour and the factors that influence both it and her desire to change. Rachel has been influenced by norms within her own family and has started to make decisions about wanting things to be different for her own son. She is very aware of the potential social and health consequences of being overweight. Rachel's self-efficacy may have been undermined by the experiences that she and family members have had in trying to change their diet and lose weight and it will be important to offer appropriate support and encouragement.

Box 4.8.4 Examples of support for Rachel through process of change.

The HV should encourage and affirm Rachel's awareness and effort without pressurising Rachel to talk about her weight/weight loss on every contact.
HV: 'You're looking well – how are things going for you?'
Might be a better way of doing this than
HV: 'How are you doing with your weight loss plan?'
The former gives the control to Rachel to talk about what she wishes to talk about.

The HV should be discerning of when the sustaining of change feels overwhelming for Rachel and offer genuine encouragement and through support and questioning return the focus to how to achieve Rachel's goals.
Rachel: 'I did well at the start and I really enjoy the classes and the people – a lot of us go to both classes – but it's been a struggle of late, my partner's shifts have changed and my mum has not been well, so I have had no-one to look after Jayden. I can take him to both classes but to be honest that makes getting there much more of a slog and if I'm tired I just can't be bothered. Also I'm worried about my mum and I have been comfort eating again. The other night I got through a sharing bag of crisps to myself and then finished off a packet of biscuits that had been opened. Back to the old Rachel – honestly I'm useless'
HV: 'You don't seem useless to me, Rachel. I'm really glad that you have enjoyed the classes and you have done really well – you look great. I'm not surprised that it is feeling so hard at present. You know, and we have talked about, how hard it is to change lifetime habits, and you have started to make those changes at one of the most demanding times of life – being a new mum!! These changes take a long time and it doesn't mean that you cannot carry on with making changes because you've had this period when it has been harder to stick at it. Have you been in touch with anyone from the group? Do you know what is wrong with your mum at present? Is there anyone else who could mind Jayden for you?'

Public Health and Health Promotion for Nurses at a Glance, First Edition. Karen Wild and Maureen McGrath.
© 2019 John Wiley & Sons Ltd. Published 2019 by John Wiley & Sons Ltd.

79

Chapter 8 Skills supporting behaviour change. Example 2: Rachel

Rachel wants to lose weight

In Chapter 2 of Unit 4 we met Rachel – a young woman who had started to speak with the Health Visitor (HV) about wanting to lose weight. Rachel is severely obese (BMI = 35) and has just given birth to Jayden, her first child. We saw in Chapter 2 that Jayden's birth has given Rachel a 'cue to action'. She wants to lose weight now – not just for herself but also for her son. We also heard Rachel say that she had been on diets all her life – without success. This indicates that her self-confidence in her ability to lose weight is low and that she may need support to develop the self-efficacy to change her behaviours in order to lose weight.

In Chapter 1 of Unit 4 we considered how important context is to behaviour and to behaviour change. Rachel's health visitor would consider a number of factors that would be important when supporting her to lose weight:

• What does Rachel mean when she says she wants to lose weight? What is her goal?
• Is Rachel really ready to make changes?
• How is Rachel intending to feed Jayden?
• What postnatal support does she have?
• Weight loss is very complex and influenced by individual microbiomes and individual physiology.
• Rachel seems to see herself as a 'failed dieter'.

Readiness to change

The COM-B model (see Chapter 4 of this unit) suggests that behaviour occurs as an interaction between three necessary conditions – capability, motivation and opportunity. Rachel seems to have the motivation to change behaviour. She lacks confidence in her own capability to make a sustained change. The HV needs to explore with her how realistic her opportunities to change are at this time. In exploring Rachel's lack of confidence the HV would firstly ask her what she means by 'losing weight' (see Box 4.8.1) and then ask her what has happened when she has tried to lose weight previously (see Box 4.8.2). These conversations enable the HV to have some initial insight into the **causality** (see Chapter 1 of this unit) of Rachel's behaviour. Rachel's norm has been to eat (and enjoy) calorie-dense foods — often high in fat and sugar, and to snack regularly between meals – particularly in the evening. Rachel eats more if she is stressed or unhappy. Her close family have the same eating pattern. Rachel has never enjoyed sports or exercise and feels at present that she could not do very much of anything 'active' because of her weight. With regard to **degree of control** over her behaviour, Rachel has had periods when she has managed to eat differently and has lost weight. She has found this difficult to sustain for any length of time. With regard to **susceptibility and risk** associated with her current behaviour Rachel is aware of the health risks associated with being overweight and says she has experienced negative comments about her weight throughout her life. She feels her weight might stop her doing some of the things she would like to do with her son. She is very keen that her son eats healthily and does not become overweight.

Support through process of readiness to change

In Chapter 4 of this unit we looked at 'readiness' being a process as well as a state. The HV would want to support Rachel to achieve the goal she has set herself of losing weight and maintaining a healthy diet for both herself and Jayden. It would be important to discuss with Rachel that this postnatal period can be demanding in relation to new responsibilities, time, changes to sleep pattern and energy levels. Rachel wants to breastfeed Jayden and so it is important that she maintains a healthy energy intake. It may be that planning to change long established eating habits at this point in time might be too difficult in the context of her adjusting to her new role as a mother responsible for a new baby. Rachel's realistic opportunities to change may be limited at this time.

One way forward might be to discuss a referral to both an exercise programme and a weight loss programme on prescription following Rachel's 6 week postnatal check with her GP. This plan would address the factors identified by Cialdini (2007; see Chapter 3 of this unit) as important for sustained behaviour change (see Box 4.8.3).

The HV would continue to support Rachel to achieve her goal whenever Rachel attended baby clinic with Jayden or on future home visits. It would be important to affirm and encourage Rachel's self-efficacy and be able to offer practical advice in relation to a healthy diet for both Rachel and Jayden. Emotional intelligence would enable the HV to discern when empathy about the difficulty of changing behaviour would be a more appropriate focus, rather than Rachel's success in relation to weight loss and increased activity. Supporting Rachel to continue to focus on change that is realistically manageable would be an important element of support as would being willing to explore ambivalence and negativity (see Box 4.8.4).

Taking account of the context of Rachel's readiness to change in this way may help any changes that are made to be more sustainable. The aims are:

• To enable Rachel to remain motivated to change.
• To develop her self-efficacy through encouraging her optimism, confidence and resourcefulness. This could all contribute to her capability and belief in herself.
• To concentrate on supporting realistic opportunities to make sustainable changes.

Rachel's growing recognition of how the changes she engages in help her to achieve some of her goals will also positively impact on motivation, self-belief and the willingness to create further opportunities to maintain behaviour changes.

9 Further examples of supporting behaviour change: Jenny, Shaheed and Deena

Box 4.9.1 MINDSPACE – Behavioural insights to health.
Source: https://assets.publishing.service.gov.uk/government/uploads/system/uploads/attachment_data/file/60524/403936_BehaviouralInsight_acc.pdf. Licensed under Open Government License, http://www.nationalarchives.gov.uk/doc/open-government-licence/version/3/.

MINDSPACE
- **Messenger** — We are heavily influenced by who communicates information
- **Incentives** — Our responses to incentives are shaped by predictable mental shortcuts such as strongly avoiding losses
- **Norms** — We are strongly influenced by what others do
- **Defaults** — We 'go with the flow' of pre-set options
- **Salience** — Our attention is drawn to what is novel and seems relevant to us
- **Priming** — Our acts are often influenced by subconscious cues
- **Affect** — Our emotional associations can powerfully shape our actions
- **Commitment** — We seek to be consistent with our public promises, and reciprocate acts
- **Ego** — We act in ways that make us feel better about ourselves

Jenny has cellulitis

Jenny is 30 years old and has a learning disability. She lives in supported living accommodation. A consistent team of three carers provide support to Jenny and her housemates at different periods throughout the day and night. Jenny fell outside about a week ago and sustained a small wound to her leg. Jenny started to complain of more pain in the affected leg two days ago. On examination the area around the healing wound was swollen, red and felt warm. Jenny said she felt well but said her leg felt too hot. Jenny's GP diagnosed cellulitis of the skin surrounding the wound and prescribed a course of antibiotics (four times a day for 7 days) and mild painkillers. He also said that Jenny should rest and elevate the leg and also keep the skin moisturised with an emollient cream. He advised regular fluids to maintain hydration. Jenny is always very restless and finds it hard to sit for longer than 10 minutes. She likes to walk outside regularly. She often leaves meals and drinks unfinished. She understands routines but takes a while to remember them and consistently work with them. Jenny hates hospitals and becomes very distressed if she has to attend, even as an outpatient. The carers discuss with the GP that it will be possible to follow his prescribed treatment in her supported living accommodation.

Things to think about (see Box 4.9.1)

It would be helpful for the carers to agree a plan of supporting Jenny through this time so that she experiences consistency in advice and help given. It may help Jenny if she is regularly reminded that her 'new' routine is important to prevent her becoming ill and needing to go into hospital. This provides a regular incentive for her to sit and elevate her leg for a period of time and also to finish her drinks. It may be important to use concrete language with Jenny and avoid terms such as 'regularly' or 'often'. So the carers may agree with Jenny that every time she has her medicine (antibiotic) she will take it sat down and drink a large glass of water with it. She can raise her leg while she is doing this. At this time her leg can be checked and also moisturised if required. As Jenny's leg starts to heal it would be important to feedback to her what a difference her actions have made and how much better her leg looks.

Dependent on Jenny's preferred communication method, resources from the CHANGE organisation may be helpful to her (www.changepeople.org).

Shaheed is diabetic

Shaheed is a 25-year-old Muslim man who has been diagnosed with diabetes over the last year. He has type 1 diabetes controlled well with insulin injections. Both he and his wife and brother have been shown how to use his insulin injection pen correctly. Shaheed is unsure how to manage his treatment during his fasting through the holy month of Ramadan. Shaheed is faced with continuing to manage his condition and fulfil his spiritual obligations as a Muslim.

Things to think about (see Box 4.9.1)

Shaheed could speak about his concerns with the Diabetes Nurse Specialist who sees him regularly, and plan how he might manage his condition during Ramadan, a couple of months before the festival begins. Some diabetics are able to observe the fast and manage their condition through changing the times and dose of insulin that they take during this period. It would be important that Shaheed and his family are able to recognise the signs and symptoms of hypoglycaemia, hyperglycaemia and dehydration and to also know what to do about them. Muslims with diabetes are encouraged to test blood glucose levels regularly during Ramadan and to ensure that they have glucose, insulin and water with them at all times. The Muslim Council of Britain and Diabetes UK provide excellent joint resources on fasting at Ramadan and are clear that anyone who is at risk of serious ill health through fasting is exempt. Shaheed and his nurse could jointly agree a plan to be shared with his local Imam, one that would aim to support him to observe the fast with clear directions of what should happen if he starts to feel unwell.

Deena wants help to stop drinking

Deena's mum had contacted the school because she was concerned about the gradual lack of social engagement Deena (aged 14) was having within the family. On a couple of occasions she had come home late from school, smelling of alcohol and behaving aggressively and out of character. Deena's mum is in the middle of a divorce from Deena's stepfather and lives alone with Deena and her younger step-sibling, who has learning difficulties. Deena has started to spend a lot of time with a group of teenagers on the estate where they live. Deena has always done well in her studies, but recently she has been failing to achieve expected grades. Last week Deena had broken down in tears in the middle of an argument with her mum and had begged her mum to help her stop drinking.

Things to think about (see Box 4.9.1)

Deena's behaviour may have been influenced by a number of life circumstances. Her mum is likely to have found it difficult to confront Deena's drinking because of her other responsibilities and it might have seemed the best option to avoid confrontation with her. She could access support from the school nurse and school staff to support her in responding to Deena's request for help. Deena seems to be at a stage where she is ready to make a change. Using some of the models of health behaviour, the School Nurse could start to explore Deena's attitude towards her drinking behaviour, the influence of subjective norms and her perceived behavioural control, enabling her to weigh up positives (fitting in with peer group) against negatives (her anger towards her family and her lack of progress at school).

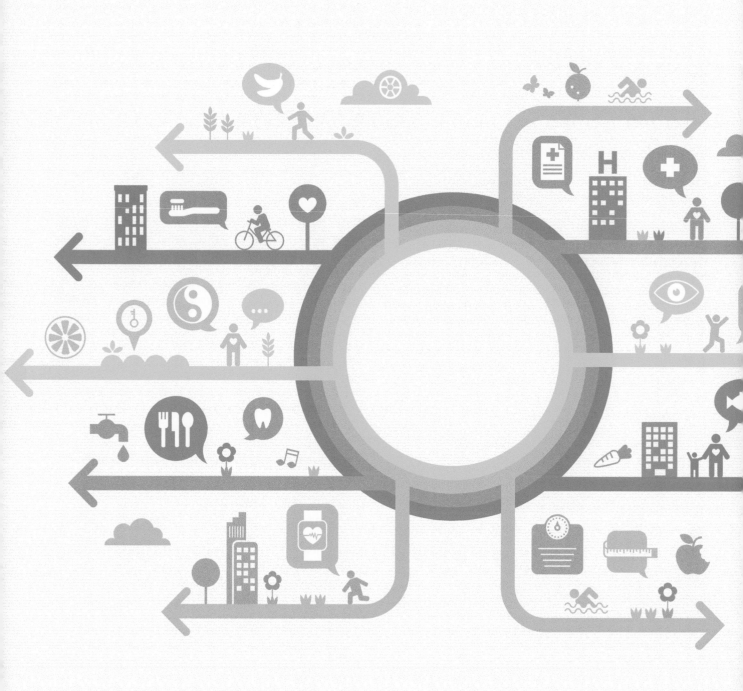

Strategies for working with communities to improve health

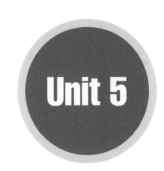

Unit 5

Chapters

Thinking points for NMC Revalidation

Looking at the community health profiles from your area, as discussed in Unit 5, what have emerged as the main reasons for morbidity and mortality in your area? How might you use this information to influence your approach to health promotion locally?

1 Community health and public health

Box 5.1.1 Ladder of interventions. Source: Nuffield Council on Bioethics (2007). Reproduced with permission of NCB.

- **Eliminate choice.** Introduce laws that entirely eliminate choice, for example compulsory isolation of people with infectious diseases.

- **Restrict choice.** Introduce laws that restrict the options available to people, for example, removing unhealthy ingredients from foods, or unhealthy foods from shops or restaurants.

- **Guide choice through disincentives.** Introduce financial or other disincentives to influence people's behaviour, for example, increasing taxes on cigarettes, or bringing in charging schemes to discourage car use in inner cities.

- **Guide choices through incentives.** Introduce financial or other incentives to influence people's behaviours, for example, offering tax-breaks on buying bicycles for travelling to work.

- **Guide choices through changing the defalut policy.** For example, changing the standard side dish restaurant from chips to a healthier alternative, with chips remaining as an option available.

- **Enable choice.** Help individuals to change their behaviours, for example, providing free 'stop smoking' programmes, building cycle lanes or providing free fruit in schools.

- **Provide information.** Inform and educate the public, for example, campaigns to encourage people to walk more or eat five portions of fruit and vegetables a day.

- **Do nothing or simply monitor the current situation.**

Public Health and Health Promotion for Nurses at a Glance, First Edition. Karen Wild and Maureen McGrath.
© 2019 John Wiley & Sons Ltd. Published 2019 by John Wiley & Sons Ltd.

Community health and population health

Nurses will in the main work with individuals when they are supporting a change in health behaviour. But it is important that nurses are aware of the factors that impact on the health of the populations and communities that these individuals are part of. It is also important for nurses to be aware of programmes that aim to mitigate the impact of factors that influence health and health behaviour. It may well be that some nurses will be involved in designing, managing and implementing programmes and interventions aimed at supporting improvement in the health of populations and communities, at some point in their careers.

Population health

Population health refers to the health of a defined population as opposed to an individual. Population may be defined by a particular indicator, for example, by gender, ethnicity or a geographical area (e.g. Salford, England, Great Britain).

Community health

Community health refers to the health of a group recognised as having a number of things in common by virtue of belonging to a specific geographical locality (wards, super-output areas) or through identification with a specific group, for example, asylum seekers, the LGBT community, nurses or Buddhists. Generally a community is more specifically defined than a population in relation to health.

Health improvement at community and population level

Much of this book has concentrated on individual health behaviours and how best to support change for an individual. It has also considered the different influences on an individual's health and how many of these influences are largely outside the control of the individual. The political, regulatory and economic environments in which people live have a significant impact on their health and the realistic choices they are able to make in respect of their health (Nuffield Council on Bioethics, 2007). Most of the improvement in mortality and morbidity in the UK through the nineteenth and twentieth centuries has been achieved through programmes, policies and interventions that are outside of medicine and the NHS. Provision of clean water, improved sanitation, and laws and regulations related to living and working environments have had the greatest impact on population health, along with the significant contribution made by vaccination programmes, screening programmes, antibiotics and other pharmacological advances.

Nurses who work with populations and communities to improve health have an important role in identifying those factors that **determine** health and result in many of the **risk factors** for health that nurses recognise in their patient assessments. For example a nurse who identifies high prevalence of risk factors for health such as hypertension, overweight or smoking in the individuals he/she meets may also recognise that some of the key determinants of health in a community are poverty, unemployment and an obesogenic environment. An individual nurse may feel unable to effect any difference to this situation but nurses can ensure that local Clinical Commissioning Groups and Health and Wellbeing Boards are made aware of health determinants that impact on populations, communities and individuals. They can also work to support advocates from local communities in lobbying local and national commissioners and politicians in order to influence the design and provision of services and environments.

Universal or targeted interventions?

Because there is good evidence on the correlation between socioeconomic status and health status at individual and community level, and on the association between income inequality and overall health status at population level (Marmot, 2010; Rowlingson, 2011) there is discussion around the need for universal interventions (aimed at everyone in a population) versus targeted interventions (aimed at the most needy). Some question the stigmatisation that may arise from targeting services to the most needy (Nuffield Council on Bioethics, 2007). There is, however, evidence that universal public health interventions can result in exacerbation of health inequalities (Blaxter, 2007; NICE, 2007, 2016).

There is also discussion about the level of intrusiveness into individual lives that public health interventions may pose. The proportionality of a public health intervention should relate to the importance of the proposed public health objectives and the likely effectiveness of the intervention. The Nuffield Council on Bioethics (2007) has developed a Ladder of Interventions (Box 5.1.1) as a way of assessing the acceptability and justification of different types of public health interventions.

Nurses should be aware of the nature of different community and population interventions aimed at improving health and should work with individuals and communities to take advantage of them in order to mitigate the impact of some of the wider determinants on their health experience and behaviours.

2 Factors that influence the health of communities

Table 5.2.1 Ten universal insights into factors that impact on people making decisions to change health-related behaviours. Source: Department of Health (2011). Licensed under Open Government Licence v3.0. http://www.nationalarchives.gov.uk/doc/open-government-licence/version/3/.

Insight	Potential leverage
People can feel powerless to change. However, if people can succeed in one area, they gain a sense of empowerment that can be used to inspire further changes	Merge databases and pursue cross-selling strategy (e.g. contact successful quitters with offers about other 'lifestyle changes)
There is a universal belief that "it will never happen to me", especially among younger people	Consider use of role models as credible witnesses
People live for today, preferring immediate benefits and discounting future negative health consequences	Develop immediate and tangible rewards and incentives
There are a small number of teachable moments associated with major lifestyle events (such as the birth of a first child; or diagnosis of a long-term condition) when people are more open to change and actively seek new information	Use the communications channels of partners and intermediaries to reach people during these moments
People seek to conform to perceived social norms and will adjust their behaviour to fit in with what they believe other people are doing	Trial communications solutions that challenge incorrect assumptions about social norms (for example that most people regularly drink more than the recommended guidelines)
People are more likely to start to modify a behaviour if they can make a series of small changes, rather than change completely	Find ways to break behaviour changes into manageable "chunks" with mechanisms for transitioning people
People are prepared to make changes for others that they would not make for their own health	Use the power of children as a motivator (and as change-agents within families)
In general, people respond to more positive, optimistic messages	Place people at the centre of their own change, rather than lecturing; continue more positive tone established by Change4Life and messages such as 'Most pregnant women do not drink alcohol' as opposed to 'Do not drink when pregnant'
People will not act if they are unsure of the outcome, or if they believe the treatment is worse than the condition	Use partners, particularly the charities, to spread good news messages (such as improved cancer survival rates) so that people can see a benefit to them in taking the first step towards action
People delay seeking help, even when they notice change, whether because they do not recognise common symptoms of illness or do not feel entitled to access services	Challenge the assumption that physical and mental deterioration is a natural part of the ageing process, or should be accepted as the cost of previous poor behaviours

Public Health and Health Promotion for Nurses at a Glance, First Edition. Karen Wild and Maureen McGrath.
© 2019 John Wiley & Sons Ltd. Published 2019 by John Wiley & Sons Ltd.

Factors that influence community health

As indicated in earlier chapters different factors combine to impact on the health of communities including:

• **Physical factors** such as access to health services, healthy foods, safe environments for physical activity, access to work, access to good education.

• **Social and cultural factors** such as a sense of 'belonging' to a community, cultural influences on diet, health behaviours, agency of individuals within a community and integration.

• **Individual behaviours,** which impact on health positively or negatively. The control that individuals have over their health may be limited in a number of ways, and people who are disadvantaged in relation to income, educational achievement and social position bear the larger burden of morbidity and early mortality in a community.

• **Community organisation** in relation to how well the community organises and works together to facilitate a health-promoting context for the individuals that live and work within it (Davies et al., 2014).

All of these factors should be taken into account when working with members of a community to support health improvement. For example, a health visitor may wish to support the parents in a community to establish a healthy weaning club to provide knowledge and ideas about when to wean and how to use affordable healthy foods to wean children on to more solid foods. The health visitor would need to take account of: availability of a safe physical space to meet; facilities to demonstrate preparation and cooking of foods; accessibility of affordable healthy foods to this community; accessibility that different families have to cooking and refrigeration/freezing facilities in their own homes; and factors that determine the types of foods purchased by people, such as when they have money available, the other children in the household, and the shelf life of the foods they purchase when they do have money available. It would be important to work closely with the parents to develop a 'club' that supported them in realistic and sustainable ways and over which they felt they had some agency and control. If these important factors are not taken account of then it is unlikely that individuals within the community will make any changes to weaning practices.

The Department of Health produced a document in 2011 ('Changing Behaviour Improving Outcomes') that identified 10 insights into key factors that influence the decisions that people make to change a health-related behaviour (Table 5.2.1). Again, it is important that nurses working with people to improve the health of communities take account of these insights.

Insights with examples

People can feel powerless to change and people are more likely to manage a series of small changes. It is important that the goals of behaviour change programmes are not set too high and where possible are individually agreed. A community mental health nurse may set up an allotment group with people from their caseload who have been diagnosed with enduring mental health problems. For some of the group the only goal set initially may be that they would agree to be accompanied to the allotment site and return home if they did not feel they could stay. 'Small successes' can encourage people to go on to develop other goals for themselves.

It will never happen to me and living for today. We have discussed in previous chapters that people are influenced by what they immediately observe about themselves and others and we could all cite behaviours that we **know** are not good for our health but which we enjoy and which we feel we can continue to indulge in with impunity as we do not seem to be suffering any adverse consequences. A practice nurse might set up a Healthy Lifestyle Intervention group for people at risk of coronary heart disease (CHD) because of a high cholesterol ratio and high triglycerides. Input to the group from someone who has developed coronary heart disease **may** be helpful to some, and the tangible reward of meeting with others who are in a similar position to themselves may provide the incentive to continue with the group and hopefully make some dietary and activity changes.

There are small number of teachable moments and people are prepared to make changes for others. Nurses need to be aware that at different stages of the life course there will be times when people are more motivated to consider health behaviour change. For example, most people will be prepared to do anything for the wellbeing of their children. Following a birth might be the time when someone makes a decision to change behaviour that impacts negatively on health. Starting work and taking on new responsibilities might be another time. Older people might want to make changes to enjoy good health in the 'third age' of life and be able to spend more time with partners/friends/grandchildren.

People seek to conform to perceived social norms and also respond to more positive messages. It is important that nurses speak to people about health behaviours in ways that accurately reflect the facts that are known and also to frame advice positively. Teenage pregnancy rates in England are falling – and it is thought that young people are more likely to use reliable contraception now than they were previously. Sexual health services for young people are also more accessible and 'young person friendly' than in the past, and in the internet age these facts are readily available to young people. The message that 'most young people who engage in sexual relationships use contraception' is normative and positive and should be accompanied by a discussion about also using protection against sexually transmitted diseases (STDs) and information on easily accessed STD screening services.

These insights can help nurses work in ways that are more likely to engage people and communities in health behaviour changes that remain sustainable.

Barriers to the success of community health improvement programmes

Table 5.3.1 Potential barriers to the success of health promotion/health improvement programmes. Source: Adapted from Hardiker *et al.*, (2009), and Franks *et al.*, (2012).

Barrier	Impact
Lack of clear aims/outcome measures	Important for participants, professionals and commissioners in terms of self-confidence, achievement and value for money
Time issues	• Unrealistic time scale for programme may mean outcomes will not be achieved • Events may be scheduled at a time that is not appropriate for the community • Professionals/volunteers/participants may not have the time required to participate
Accessibility problems	People may not engage if the personal, social and cultural context of the community has not been taken into account
Lack of awareness of programme	• Community cannot engage in a programme that it is unaware of • Staff/volunteers cannot successfully run a programme without being aware of all aspects of programme and their responsibilities within it • Other professionals and third sector organisations cannot signpost people to a programme that they are either not aware of or do not know the details of
Poor planning and organisation	All of the following will impact on the success of a programme: • lack of leadership • lack of resources • lack of skills in health promotion • lack of workforce stability • lack of partnership working (with community and other stakeholders) • unrealistic schedules

Approaches to engaging people in health improvement/health promotion programmes

In England Clinical Commissioning Groups (CCGs) are responsible for assessing the local health needs of the population in a defined geographical area and for securing services that address identified needs. The commissioning process is an ongoing one that responds to changing needs and assesses the success of services in addressing identified need. In the main CCGs are co-terminus with local authority areas (local authorities are now responsible for public health) and these two organisations work closely together through Health and Wellbeing Boards to generate a Joint Strategic Needs Assessment and a Health and Wellbeing Strategy. It is important that nurses contribute to both of these processes and are involved in developing and implementing programmes to address local needs.

It is important that health promotion/health improvement programmes have clearly developed aims and outcome measures in order to be able to demonstrate the success of a programme or to identify why proposed outcomes were not achieved. A comprehensive synthesis of public health interventions/programmes was completed in 2009 (Hardiker et al., 2009; Franks et al., 2012). This synthesis took account of grey literature (in the sense of reports/evaluations/audits of programmes that had been completed by local practitioners but had not been published) and so accessed useful information related to the success/failure of programmes.

In general programmes seek to engage people in behaviour change using one or more of four approaches:

- **Involvement in practical activities,** such as cooking, physical exercise, art and crafts, music, meditation.
- **Provision of advice and information** to increase knowledge and understanding, such as health cafes, wellbeing courses.
- **Improvement of access to sources,** such as staying well at work, mobile 'not-for-profit' grocery van, food cooperatives, involvement in an allotment.
- **Support and encouragement to make changes** – this is an important aspect of any programme and intended sources of support should be identified and may include professionals, peers and families.

Barriers to the success of programmes

(Table 5.3.1)

Time issues

Health promotion programmes rely on people from the relevant community finding the time to engage in activities or attend advice sessions. They also rely (certainly in the period of establishment and often for much longer) on professionals being able to regularly commit time to the programme. If either the community or the professionals cannot commit time to the programme it is likely to be less successful. The time when a programme runs also will impact on people's engagement with it. Programmes aimed at parents that run at times when other children need to be met from school will be less successful. Programmes that run during festival times may well limit the attendance by certain cultural groups. A mobile 'fruit and veg' van that visits areas on an ad hoc basis, or at times when people may not have money, will be less successful. Thought should also be given to the required duration of a programme before there can be realistic expectation that some of the planned outcomes might have been achieved. Many programmes receive funding for too short a time in which to do this.

Accessibility problems

It is important that programmes do not fail to engage with communities because of accessibility issues. The context of the community in which the programme is delivered must be taken account of. Do people have transport in the area? Is the area socially cohesive with support in terms of child care or family encouragement? Do people have good levels of literacy and numeracy? Is the area diverse in terms of culture and spoken/written language skills? Do people feel safe to go out at all times of day? Do people function better at certain times of the day. Aspects of all of these issues have been cited as reasons why people do not engage with programmes.

Lack of awareness of programme by all relevant stakeholders

If people from the community are unaware of the programme then they will not engage with it. Also if professionals/voluntary sector workers are unaware of the programme they will not signpost people to it or may do so only once people have reached crisis point.

Poor planning and organisation

Previous units and chapters have addressed the difficulty of engaging in and sustaining behaviour change. If people make a commitment to engage with a programme that supports them to make some changes/learn more about living a healthy lifestyle that is an enormous step to have made. If they then experience issues, such as turning up to a session to find it has been cancelled, being promised an 'exercise buddy' who does not materialise, waiting half an hour for a grocery van that does not turn up, they are likely to experience real discouragement. These issues can unintentionally convey the message that 'you are not important enough for us to provide this service to'. Such experiences can make people wary of engaging in any future programmes

When planning and delivering programmes that aim to support a community in addressing a health need it is important that the potential barriers to success discussed above are taken account of and that strategies are developed that will mitigate the impact of them. The next chapter will look at this when considering factors that promote the success of programmes.

Factors that may promote the success of community health improvement programmes

Table 5.4.1 Factors that may promote the success of community health improvement programmes. Source: Adapted from Hardiker et al., (2009), and Franks et al., (2012).

Promoting factor	Impact
Partnership working	• Planning, delivering and evaluating programmes in partnership with the community addresses some of identified barriers related to time and accessibility issues • People are more likely to engage with interventions that they have some sense of ownership over • People may relate well to facilitators who are from the community and who may be perceived as 'one of us'
Use of practical interventions	• Can offer more immediate and tangible evidence of 'success' • May encourage more sustained engagement, which may result in measurable health outcomes
Nature of programme	• Less formal and more flexible programmes engage people • Programmes that are designed in this way will be able to respond to changed needs throughout the process of behaviour change
Good planning and organisation	• Involvement of ALL stakeholders from the beginning of the planning stage addresses the identified barrier of lack of awareness • Clear processes of referral, links to other services and evaluation enable the capture of both intended and unintended outcome measures relevant to the community and to commissioners • The above processes enable commissioners to feel confident about sustaining the programme over a longer period of time

Public Health and Health Promotion for Nurses at a Glance, First Edition. Karen Wild and Maureen McGrath.
© 2019 John Wiley & Sons Ltd. Published 2019 by John Wiley & Sons Ltd.

Successful health improvement/health promotion in communities

In the previous chapter a number of factors were considered as potential barriers to the success of health promotion/health improvement programmes in communities. These programmes would be identified as part of a Health and Wellbeing Strategy aimed at addressing need identified in the Joint Strategic Needs Assessment. The best needs assessments always incorporate the 'voice' of the people living in a community captured through surveys, interviews, focus groups and so forth.

It is also important to engage with a community **before** a proposed intervention is planned in any detail and before it is delivered. Hardiker et al. (2009) found that interventions planned and delivered in partnership with the community were likely to be more successful in improving the health of that community. This is probably the single most important promoter of the success of a programme. Working in this way is likely to address some of the identified barriers associated with time issues and accessibility to the events and interventions associated with the programme. If people from the community help to plan the programme they will bring knowledge of personal, social and cultural contexts that professionals may not be aware of. This aids the planning of realistic programmes that are meaningful to the community who will be engaging in them.

The other key issue in relation to the success of a programme is a clear and sustained commitment to fund the programme. There should be agreement on a realistic timetable for producing health outcomes that can be quantitatively or qualitatively measured. Many interventions are funded for short periods of time such as 3–6months. Given the complexity of changing health behaviours it is not realistic to assess change in health behaviour over this period of time.

Factors promoting the success of programmes (Table 5.4.1)

Partnership working

As indicated above, planning and delivering programmes in partnership with the community is more likely to result in health improvement of that community. Engaging facilitators who are members of the community has been shown to promote success. A healthy cooking group led by people who live in the community may be helpful in encouraging people to try different foods. These facilitators would know how to budget and where to access cheap healthier foods locally. They may represent social proof to the members of the group (see Unit 4 Chapter 3) in that they may see the facilitators as 'someone like us'. Programmes that can run for long enough to enable professionals to withdraw from leadership roles and hand these over to community members are also more sustainable in the longer term. People are more likely to engage with programmes for which the community has a sense of ownership.

Use of practical activities

Interventions that involve practical activities, for example cooking, music, creating art, walking, gardening and meditating, are often more successful at engaging people over a period of time. This may be because they offer more immediate and tangible evidence of 'success' for participants in that something is produced or achieved. As engagement continues the health benefits of increased self-confidence, stress reduction and feeling more healthy may become apparent and may be eventually measurable as weight loss, reduced blood pressure reduced score on depression/anxiety scales.

Nature of programme

Programmes that are less formal and are flexible enough to respond to different individual needs are likely to be more successful and maximise participant engagement. This of course has implications for the training and skills development of people leading and delivering the programme and for the ways in which these skills are developed amongst community members who may eventually deliver the programme. This factor is important. If people are engaging in programmes that support behaviour change their needs will be different as they begin to make changes.

Good planning and organisation

Programmes can be flexible and informal and still be well organised. Those designing and implementing programmes should from the beginning of the planning process engage with the community, with professionals working in the community, with third sector organisations in the community and with the commissioners of the programme. This helps to ensure that programmes are directly relevant to the community and realistic in terms of outcomes. This also ensures that all relevant stakeholders are aware of the programme right from the start and that marketing of the programme to the community is appropriate in relation to factors such as culture, age and language.

Where possible and appropriate there should be plans to incorporate successful programmes into established mainstream services so that they can be sustained in the future.

Programmes should have clear referral processes, planned exit routes and links to other programmes, and should use a range of evaluation methods to capture both intended and unintended outcome measures. These can be creatively designed to work with programmes that need to have elements of flexibility and informality.

Staff involved in planning and delivering programmes should have appropriate skills, ongoing training and sustained organisational support.

Working as part of a successful health promotion programme can be extremely demanding but can also be one of the most rewarding roles a nurse undertakes.

5 Health profiles

Figure 5.5.1 A variety of different profiles are available for all local authority areas in England and are updated regularly. Examples of the health profiles are illustrated here. Source: Public Health England. Licensed under Open Government Licence v3.0. http://www.nationalarchives.gov.uk/doc/open-government-licence/version/3/.

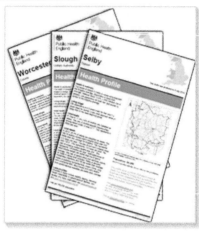

Figure 5.5.2 An illustration of a mental health profile. Source: Public Health England. Licensed under Open Government Licence v3.0. http://www.nationalarchives.gov.uk/doc/open-government-licence/version/3/.

Wider determinants of health

The wider determinants have been described as the causes of the causes. They are the social, economic and environmental conditions that influence the health of individuals and populations. They determine the extent to which a person has the right physical, social and personal resources to achieve their goals, meet needs and deal with changes to their circumstances.

		Local value	Eng. value	Eng. worst*	England Range	Eng. Best*
1	Percentage of 16–18 year olds not in employment, education or training, 2011	7.3	6.2	11.9		1.9
2	Episodes of violent crime, rate per 1,000 population, 2010/11	16.8	14.6	34.5		6.3
3	Percentage of the relevant population living in the 20% most deprived areas in England, 2010	44.6	19.8	83.0		0.3
4	Working age adults who are unemployed, rate per 1,000 population, 2010/11	84.3	59.4	105.2		8.3
5	Rate of hospital admissions for alcohol attributable conditions, per 1,000 population, 2011/12	32.5	23.0	38.6		11.4
6	Numbers of people (aged 18–75) in drug treatment, rate per 1,000 population, 2011/12	13.0	5.2	0.8		18.4

Risk factors

A risk factor is any attribute, characteristic or exposure of an individual that increases the likelihood of developing a disease, injury or mental health problem. Some examples of the more important risk factors in mental health are under and over weight, low levels of physical activity, drug abuse, tobacco and alcohol consumption, and homelessness.

		Local value	Eng. value	Eng. worst*	England Range	Eng. Best*
7	Statutory homeless households, rate per 1,000 households, all ages, 2010/11	0.38	2.03	10.36		0.13
8	Percentage of the population with a limiting long term illness, 2001	23.1	16.9	24.4		10.2
9	First time entrants into the youth justice system 10 to 17 year olds, 2001 to 2011	1,055	876	2,435		34.3
10	Percentage of adults (15+) participating in recommended level or physical activity, 2009/10 to 2011/12	10.0	11.2	5.7		17.3

Levels of mental health and illness

At any one time, roughly one in six of us is experiencing a mental health problem, mental health problems are also estimated to cost the economy £105 billion per year it's important to monitor and investigate the levels of mental health in order to target and improve mental health services at a local level.

		Local value	Eng. value	Eng. worst*	England Range	Eng. Best*
11	Percentage of adults (18+) with dementia, 2011/12	0.54	0.53	0.95		0.21
12	Ratio of recorded to expected prevalence of dementia, 2010/11	0.44	0.42	0.27		0.69
13	Percentage of adults (18+) with depression, 2011/12	10.49	11.68	20.29		4.75
14	Percentage of adults (18+) with learning disability, 2011/12	0.67	0.45	0.21		0.77

The purpose of health profiling

Profiles of the health of a population enable information about health, and the determinants of health, in relation to a population/community to be collated. This information can then be analysed and used to inform strategies aimed at improving the health of that population. It is important that any profiling process takes account of the views of the people who make up that population as well as statistical information collected from local authority and health services. A profile may indicate rates of prevalence for long-term/enduring mental health issues collected from GPs as part of the Quality and Outcomes Framework (https://qof.digital.nhs.uk/). It would also be important to directly access the views of the population in relation to how many would report that they viewed themselves as living with long-term mental health problems and look further into what this meant for them in their daily lives and for their general health.

Sources of health profile information

At a local level the Joint Strategic Needs Assessments and Health and Wellbeing Strategies mentioned in Chapter 3 of this unit are made available on the websites of all local authorities, and these are increasingly incorporating the qualitative work that accesses patients' reported views on their own health. For nurses who are involved in strategies aimed at working with a community it is important that they contribute to and use these local documents to inform their work. All nurses can gain a great deal through being aware of sources of health profiling related to the people who live in the area in which they work. Hospital nurses need to know the context from which their patients have entered hospital and will return to on discharge. This will enable work with patients to be more meaningful and relevant when used in individual nurse-patient relationships.

There are also very useful open access sources on health in relation to specific geographical areas, which can be accessed via the NHS UK Hospital Episode Statistics site (https://content.digital.nhs.uk/hes) and the Public Health Profiles site (https://fingertips.phe.org.uk/) held by Public Health England. This latter site consists of a range of different profiles related to general health, children and young people's health, mental health and learning disability (see Figures 5.5.1 and 5.5.2). There are also profiles related to particular conditions and health indicators such as cardiovascular disease, cancers, lung conditions, sexual and reproductive health, depression, dementia, physical activity, tobacco control and oral health. The site has also started to publish profiles in relation to factors that impact on general health such as antimicrobial resistance and adult social care. It is possible to 'drill down' and locate information in relation to specific indicators at local authority level. As mentioned in Chapter 3 of this unit, most local authority and Clinical Commissioning Group areas are co-terminus and so this is very useful information for the development of strategies to improve health within communities.

The Public Health Profiles information is updated yearly and allows prevalence comparison of all health indicators at regional and England levels, which makes health inequalities across regions and across England transparent.

We would recommend that you access the Public Health Profiles website and access the profile that is relevant to your clinical speciality and geographical area of practice. Think about how the information that you access could be used to improve the health of the patient group you have most contact with.

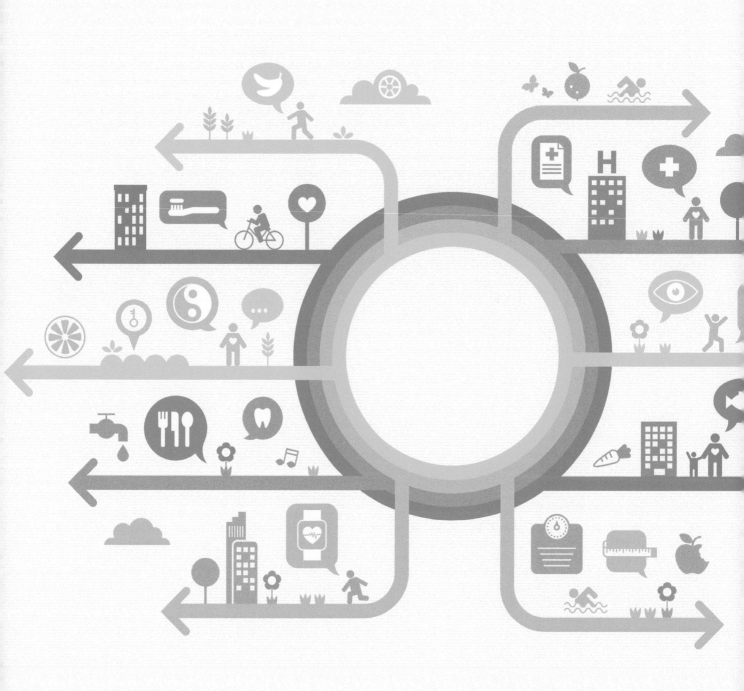

Ethics of public health and health promotion

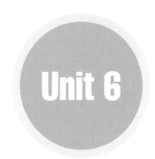

Unit 6

Thinking points for NMC Revalidation

On completion of Unit 6 we invite you to select one of the ethical principles. Think about how this impacts upon your care. What rights do your patients have in relation to this principle and health promotion?

1   Ethical principles

Figure 6.1.1 Ethical principles.

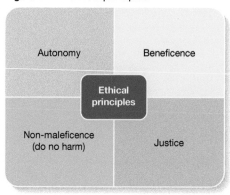

Autonomy

Beneficence

Ethical principles

Non-maleficence (do no harm)

Justice

Table 6.1.1 Three types of justice associated with the care setting.

Egalitarian justice	Concerned with the distribution of health-care resources in accordance with individual need. In this perspective individual need should be met by equal access to services
Libertarian justice	This perspective relates to liberty and choice and is associated with how hard an individual has worked in order to earn health care; they are judged on merit
Rights-based justice	Implies that the state has an obligation to provide care and that the patient should suffer no harm as a result of that provision. People's rights have to be upheld in order to meet the criteria associated with a rights perspective

Public Health and Health Promotion for Nurses at a Glance, First Edition. Karen Wild and Maureen McGrath.
© 2019 John Wiley & Sons Ltd. Published 2019 by John Wiley & Sons Ltd.

Ethics is relevant to all areas of health-care practice, and the wider aspects of research, management and education fall under this umbrella. Active involvement in ethical decision-making is an integral part of public health, not least because the primary aims of health care are to do good and to minimise harm. These two fundamental considerations when engaging in public health are significant overarching ethical principles, and are linked together with justice and the belief in a person's individual rights. There are four principles (Figure 6.1.1) and these are applied to ethics in the wider context. Not to be confused with ethical issues, the four principles are:

- Autonomy
- Beneficence
- Non-maleficence
- Justice.

Autonomy

The term 'autonomy' is derived from the Greek and is broadly defined as self-determination or self-rule, and focuses on the ability to make one's own decisions and have the right to choose. It recognises the uniqueness of individuals and that the person has the right to self-determination. Choice is effective if knowledge and understanding of what is possible exists. From a public health perspective, minimising ill health is an important goal towards maximising personal autonomy. Health education promotes awareness, thus enabling autonomous behaviour.

Beneficence

The principle of 'doing good' in a health-care context can be linked to a duty to avoid doing harm. Health-care practitioners have an obligation to do good for patients and individuals in their care and to support and act in a way that benefits individuals or groups. It can be argued then that beneficence is a duty of care.

Non-maleficence

Non-maleficence means to 'do no harm' and works with the principle of beneficence. At face value, this seems a simple mantra to follow, but in reality it can be complicated. Practitioners should never intentionally cause harm. Beauchamp and Childress (2009) point out the difficulty in defining the nature of harm. There are many types, ranging from physical and emotional injury to deprivation of property or violation of rights. In health care, harm can have a narrower definition, including pain, disability, emotional harm or death. Harm is a subjective entity and can mean different things to different people. Harm may have to be accepted in order to bring about good, for example administering painful injections to deliver life-saving medications.

Justice

Justice is often referred to as fairness, and being fair and right is something most people would aim for. Patients may be forgiven for asking the question 'Is it fair that I have to wait for this or that treatment?' When justice is discussed in a health-care arena, there are many factors that will influence whether we are being fair and right. Table 6.1.1 identifies the three perspectives associated with justice within the care setting.

Other terms that are associated with justice are:

- Justice as a means of punishment or retribution (an eye for an eye). Punishment or retribution has more to do with the law than health. Crime is punishable by society through the judicial system.
- Justice as fairness (fair distribution).
- Justice as entitlement.

In defining the term justice, Beauchamp and Childress (2009) suggest that justice is the fair, equitable and appropriate treatment of all people. The underpinning principle associated with justice, therefore, is that everyone is valued equally and treated alike. Being fair and equitable will also depend on what society feels is owed to others – it is therefore subjective and can be loaded with values and judgements. Justice to individuals also implies care that does not discriminate on the basis of sexual orientation, gender, race, religion, age or illness (physical and psychological).

2 Nursing and ethics

Box 6.2.1 Professional standards for practice and behaviour for nurses and midwives.
Source: NMC (2015) The Code: *Professional standards of practice and behaviour for nurses and midwives.*

The Code (NMC, 2015) contains a series of statements that taken together signify what good nursing and midwifery practice looks like. It puts the interests of patients and service users first, is safe and effective, and promotes trust through professionalism.

Prioritise people

- Treat people as individuals and uphold their dignity.
- Listen to people and respond to their preferences and concerns.
- Make sure that people's physical, social and psychological needs are assessed and responded to.
- Act in the best interests of people at all times.
- Respect people's right to privacy and confidentiality.

Practise effectively

- Always practise in line with the best available evidence.
- Communicate clearly.
- Work cooperatively.
- Share your skills, knowledge and experience for the benefit of people receiving care and your colleagues.
- Keep clear and accurate records relevant to your practice.
- Be accountable for your decisions to delegate tasks and duties to other people.
- Have in place an indemnity arrangement which provides appropriate cover for any practice you take on as a nurse or midwife in the United Kingdom.

Preserve safety

- Recognise and work within the limits of your competence.
- Be open and candid with all service users about all aspects of care and treatment, including when any mistakes or harm have taken place.
- Always offer help if an emergency arises in your practice setting or anywhere else.
- Act without delay if you believe that there is a risk to patient safety or public protection.
- Raise concerns immediately if you believe a person is vulnerable or at risk and needs extra support and protection.
- Advise on, prescribe, supply, dispense or administer medicines within the limits of your training and competence, the law, our guidance and other relevant policies, guidance and regulations.
- Be aware of, and reduce as far as possible, any potential for harm associated with your practice.

Promote professionalism and trust

- Uphold the reputation of your profession at all times.
- Uphold your position as a registered nurse or midwife.
- Fulfil all registration requirements.
- Cooperate with all investigations and audits.
- Respond to any complaints made against you professionally.
- Provide leadership to make sure people's wellbeing is protected and to improve their experiences of the health-care system.

Nursing ethics

Nursing practice is structured by codes of ethics and standards (shown in Box 6.2.1) that are intended to guide nursing practice and to protect the public. Individual nursing practice can be held to these standards in a court of law. The guidelines are especially important because nurses encounter legal and ethical problems almost daily. The large number of ethical issues facing nurses within clinical practice makes the standards for nurses and midwives critical to moral and ethical decision-making. These standards also help to define the roles of nurses.

Professional nursing organisations develop and implement standards of practice to help clarify the nurse's responsibilities to society. In the UK, the Nursing and Midwifery Council (NMC, 2015) identifies standards of conduct (as set out in Box 6.2.1). It also identifies standards of performance and ethics for nurses and midwives.

Public Health and Health Promotion for Nurses at a Glance, First Edition. Karen Wild and Maureen McGrath.
© 2019 John Wiley & Sons Ltd. Published 2019 by John Wiley & Sons Ltd.

One of the key components for measuring competency in nursing is the application and delivery of ethical practice and care. This recognises that an established code of ethics is one criterion that defines a profession, and acknowledges that an ethical code is an essential feature of nursing care. Ethics are principles of conduct, and ethical behaviour is concerned with values, moral duty, obligations and the distinction between right and wrong. There are a number of approaches that can be considered.

Applied ethics

Applied ethics is the term used to describe an approach to ethical decision-making that uses moral theories and principles to examine and address practical issues in everyday professional life. This approach acknowledges that ethics are not just about the big issues, such as life and death. In nursing, everyday approaches to care should reflect an ethical stance. Just as nurses are encouraged to reflect on the care that they deliver, they are also encouraged to reflect ethically on actions that they engage in on an ongoing basis.

Applied ethics help us to find the moral ground from which we can view the issues in public life. They help us to identify morally correct approaches (and therefore support nurses in recognising when actions are not ethical) in the care environment.

There are three common approaches to the process of ethical thinking:

1 Rules-based (deontology)
2 Outcomes-based (utilitarian)
3 Virtue-based.

Deontology

Rules-based ethics are often described as 'duty-based' and are concerned with the idea that some acts are right and some are wrong. As a result of this, people have a duty to act accordingly, regardless of the consequences of the act; whether an action is ethical depends on the intentions behind the decisions, rather than the outcomes. Deontological ethics (deontology) considers what actions are right, and has fundamental moral rules, such as: it is wrong to kill, to steal and to tell lies, and it is right to keep promises.

Generally, deontologists are bound by constraints, for example the prerequisite not to kill, but they are also given options, for example the right not to donate money to a charity if they do not wish to. There are, however, complexities to the notion of deontology, because ideas of duty and what is right can vary among individuals from various cultural backgrounds.

Strict utilitarians, in contrast, recognise neither constraints nor options, and the aim of the utilitarian is to maximise the good by any and all means necessary.

Outcomes-based ethics – utilitarianism

A useful way of describing the utilitarian perspective is 'the greatest good for the greatest number' – this can be interpreted as always acting in such a way that will produce the greatest overall amount of good in the world. The value of the act is determined by its usefulness, with the main emphasis on the outcome or consequence. The focus or the moral position arising from utilitarianism is to put aside our own self-interests for the sake of all. It is often referred to as consequentialism, and is based on the notion that in ethical decision-making, the person should choose the action that maximises good consequences. If a nurse uses a utilitarian approach with regard to truth telling for example, he/she would have to take into account, when making a decision, the consequence or the outcome of truth telling, and whether the act (telling the truth) would produce more happiness than unhappiness. In this circumstance, even if a decision is made to tell the truth in order to arrive at the greatest good for the greatest number, this may not necessarily be the morally correct theory to justify the action, a deontological approach may prove to be more appropriate.

The attraction of a utilitarian approach within large organisations such as the NHS lies in its ability to apply the greatest benefits to the greatest numbers, that is to address the health needs of the majority of the population. This can be problematic as it does not necessarily allow for individual differences. An example of this may be the need for treatment of a rare condition, which may not be included in the resource allocation that is geared to the more common health problems.

Virtue ethics

The ideology behind virtue ethics lies in the idea that it is person-based rather than action-based; it is not so much about what you should do but more focused on how you should be. Thus, it is not the consequences of actions or the duties and rules that govern actions, but rather the moral character of the person carrying out the actions that is important. The great philosophers such as Plato and Aristotle would ponder over how a virtuous person would act in certain circumstances to draw conclusions about the nature of moral behaviour.

The traditional list of cardinal virtues includes: prudence, justice, bravery and self-control. However, simply adopting these virtues to behave in an ethical way is criticised because, although it sends out positive messages about how to be a good person, it does not provide clear guidance on what to do in certain situations where dilemmas occur.

Morals and ethics

Nursing ethics is about asking ourselves whether something that can be done should be done or should not be done. Some answers can be considered more socially or morally acceptable than others, depending on the context in which they exist. When applied to the care setting, this subconscious decision-making can be influenced by our opinions and personal values, a sense of what is right or wrong, our understanding of our obligations and duties as a nurse, and the subsequent consequences of our actions. Normative ethics is the branch of philosophy that studies morality in this sense.

Just as an individual has values, it is sensible to assume that he or she will have some kind of moral code underpinning behaviour. The complexity of moral development, the means of learning what is right and wrong and what should or should not happen, begins in childhood and continues through life. An example of a moral code is the 'golden rule' that is a common message in religious texts throughout the ages: that of treating others as you would want to be treated yourself.

Morals can be thought of as standards of conduct that reflect ideal human behaviour; for example, an expectation that in society, truth and honesty will apply to all situations, regardless of negative consequences. In nursing this can be challenging; however, an insight into the ethical principles and how these relate to nursing ethical frameworks can guide nurses in difficult moral situations (Peate and Wild 2018).

3 Application of ethical principles to public health issues

Figure 6.3.1 The diversity of ethical considerations in public health.

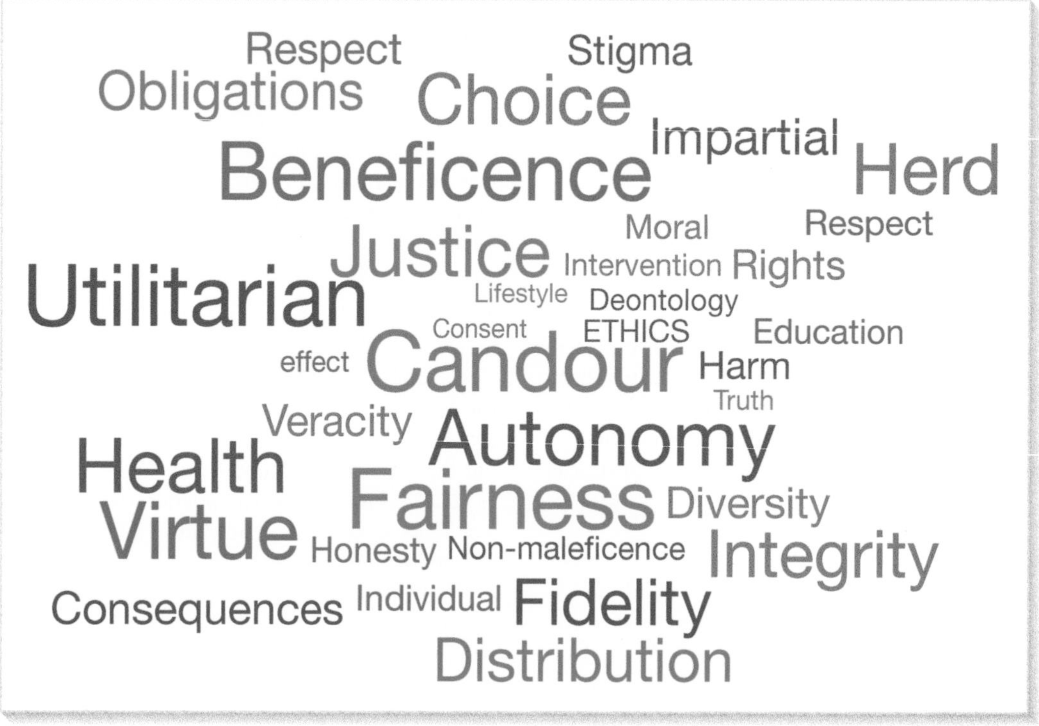

Respect Stigma
Obligations Choice
Beneficence Impartial Herd
Justice Moral Respect
Utilitarian Intervention Rights
Lifestyle Deontology
Consent ETHICS Education
effect Candour Harm
Veracity Truth
Health Autonomy
Virtue Fairness Diversity
Honesty Non-maleficence Integrity
Consequences Individual Fidelity
Distribution

Table 6.3.1 Ethical principles and approaches and examples of public health measures.

	Utilitarian	Deontological
Beneficence	Herd immunisation	
Non-maleficence		Seat belt legislation
Autonomy	Cervical screening	
Justice	Childsmile Scotland	

Public Health and Health Promotion for Nurses at a Glance, First Edition. Karen Wild and Maureen McGrath.
© 2019 John Wiley & Sons Ltd. Published 2019 by John Wiley & Sons Ltd.

Autonomy

Freedom of choice can only be exercised where choice exists, and from a public health perspective this means that the information is readily available from which choices can be informed. Thus individuals may choose healthy options/lifestyles based on an understanding of those choices. In health promotion, where the goal is to encourage healthy habits, barriers to choice can exist. For instance, obesity prevention campaigns could stigmatise the persons affected if they represent individuals as being exclusively responsible for dietary habits – the so-called 'victim blaming' – that are in great measure determined by social, economic, genetic and cultural factors outside the control of the individual. In an ideal world, a competent person might be encouraged to act in a way that would benefit health by:

- Receiving easily understood information about the relationship between health and lifestyle.
- The consequences to future health versus behaviour.
- Freedom of choice based on individual preferences.

In reality, individual decisions and autonomy are difficult to achieve because internal and external influences may be at odds with health promotion and education. Influences such as the environment in which one lives may make ideal choices difficult. Internal locus of control, the inability to foresee consequences and individual beliefs all play a part in the application of autonomy.

Beneficence and non-maleficence: the principles of doing good and avoiding harm

No health intervention, including a preventive or health promotion intervention, is risk-free. Whilst the harm caused to participants by public health interventions might be minimal, the impact can be extremely relevant, since such interventions tend to be targeted at a very large number of persons, most of whom are healthy. This combined with the ethical approach of utilitarian ethics (where the greatest good to the greatest number ideal applies) can help to explain or justify the possible harm caused by, for example, the 'herd effect' of vaccination programmes. Table 6.3.1 demonstrates how principles and approaches like this can work together. For example, immunisation programmes aim to protect large numbers from disease with minimal risk to individuals.

Justice

A stance taken by the Scottish Parliament is to apply elements of Social Justice into their distribution of health care. The recognition that the surest way to reduce health inequalities might be to stop trying to improve the health of the well off is applied in dental health care. Dental care reaches the most affluent in the most effective way, therefore widening inequalities. As such, the 'Childsmile' scheme (Shaw et al., 2009) seeks to target dental health to lower socioeconomic groups by:

- The distribution of free toothbrushes, fluoride toothpaste, and a feeding cup via health visitors and nurseries.
- Referral of families at risk via the health visitor to dental health support workers, dental nurses, and dental practices.
- Nursery/school initiatives with twice yearly fluoride varnish and fissure sealants applied to children's teeth, and ongoing oral health promotion.

4 The stewardship model

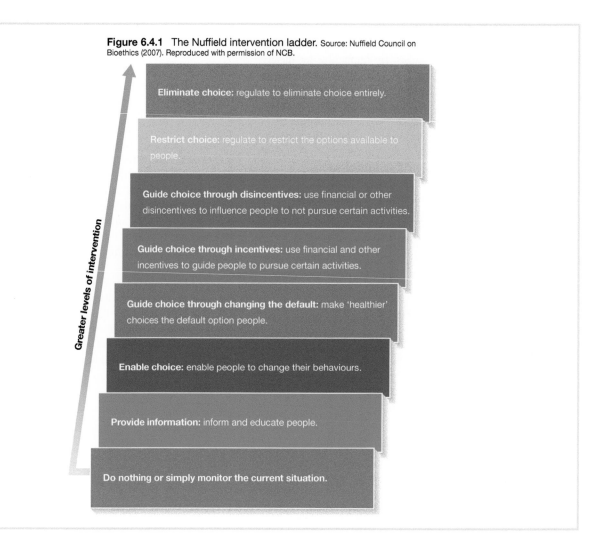

Figure 6.4.1 The Nuffield intervention ladder. Source: Nuffield Council on Bioethics (2007). Reproduced with permission of NCB.

Greater levels of intervention

Eliminate choice: regulate to eliminate choice entirely.

Restrict choice: regulate to restrict the options available to people.

Guide choice through disincentives: use financial or other disincentives to influence people to not pursue certain activities.

Guide choice through incentives: use financial and other incentives to guide people to pursue certain activities.

Guide choice through changing the default: make 'healthier' choices the default option people.

Enable choice: enable people to change their behaviours.

Provide information: inform and educate people.

Do nothing or simply monitor the current situation.

Public Health and Health Promotion for Nurses at a Glance, First Edition. Karen Wild and Maureen McGrath.
© 2019 John Wiley & Sons Ltd. Published 2019 by John Wiley & Sons Ltd.

If we accept the notion that public health places an emphasis on health improvement and prevention of ill health, then we ought to make provision for the sorts of measures that will protect and promote the best health outcomes possible. However, some public health measures can be seen to restrict personal freedom and choice. Measures such as the smoking ban in public places, alcohol licensing and food labelling can be regarded by some as examples of a 'nanny state' where there is a so-called unnecessary intrusion into people's lives and what they do, eat and drink. The counter argument would suggest that government intervention can safeguard public health. Deciding what type of measure will be appropriate and effective has long been a problem for policy makers. Legislation brings about changes, and sets new standards for the public good. This kind of approach is a form of 'stewardship'.

Fundamental to the notion of stewardship is the question 'whose responsibility is health?' Autonomy to adopt healthy lifestyles should be a simple assumption, but the notion of 'choice' can be problematic, as choices are often inhibited by the actions of others, and by intrinsic and extrinsic factors affecting health, such as socioeconomic, environmental and genetic factors.

Balancing individual freedom with community benefits has been a longstanding ethical dilemma in public health and traditional bioethics. Some measures in public health policy can impose minor violations of individual freedom for the greater good. The Nuffield Council on Bioethics (2007) produced a report that challenged this balance and produced a model for public health ethics. This model, known as the 'stewardship model' (described more fully in Chapter 5 of this unit), outlines a framework of responsibilities that so-called liberal governments have towards the population, those of unnecessary coercion and restriction of freedom. In addition, 'stewardship' recognises that governments have a duty to reduce inequality, provide healthy options and to protect the health of the most vulnerable in society

The stewardship model was proposed as a basis for making decisions about public health issues including alcohol and tobacco, infectious diseases, obesity and water fluoridation in the Council's 2007 report, Public Health: Ethical Issues. Killoran and White (2007) address the stewardship model as '[defining] appropriate means of achieving public health goals that are highly relevant to NICE's purpose:
* promoting health through programmes to support behaviour change as well as providing information and advice
* aiming to ensure that it is easy for people to lead a healthy life through changes in the physical and social environment
* ensuring that people have access to medical services and addressing health inequalities.'

The 'intervention ladder'

Aligned to the stewardship approach (and helpful in translating the somewhat philosophical model) is the 'intervention ladder'. This is a tool that enables the ranking of public health measures according to their coerciveness or intrusiveness. Figure 6.4.1 shows the different stages or rungs to the ladder, which range from at the very lowest level 'do nothing', to the top rung, which asserts the need to eliminate choice. The higher up the ladder an intervention ranks, the stronger the need for justification and sound evidence for implementation. An example of a measure at the top of the ladder might be an outbreak of Ebola. Compulsory quarantine or isolation clearly involves a significant infringement of liberty. The suggestion is that these measures may be ethically justified where the harm to others can be significantly reduced, a clear example of utilitarian ethics.

5 Acceptable health goals

Figure 6.5.1 The stewardship model.

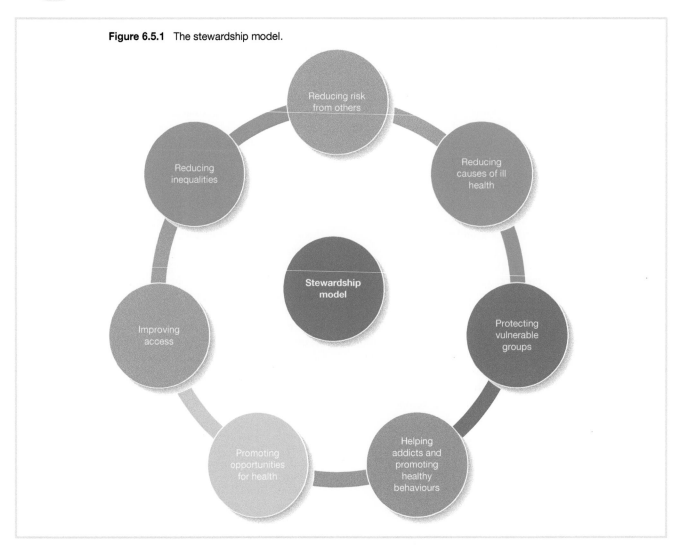

The 'stewardship model'

The Nuffield Council on Bioethics (2007) starts from the position

that the state has a duty to enable people to lead healthy lives. Everyone should have a fair opportunity to lead a healthy life, and therefore governments should try to remove inequalities that affect disadvantaged groups or individuals. We propose a 'stewardship model' that outlines the ethical principles that should be considered by public health policy makers.

Figure 6.5.1 provides an overview of the stewardship model to enable the reader to understand the approaches that can support public health goals.

Acceptable public health goals include:

- Reducing the risks of ill health that result from other people's actions, such as drink-driving and smoking in public places.
- Reducing causes of ill health relating to environmental conditions, for instance provision of clean drinking water and setting housing standards.
- Protecting and promoting the health of children and other vulnerable people.
- Helping people to overcome addictions that are harmful to health or helping them to avoid unhealthy behaviours.
- Ensuring that it is easy for people to lead a healthy life, for example by providing convenient and safe opportunities for exercise.
- Ensuring that people have appropriate access to medical services.
- Reducing unfair health inequalities.

At the same time, public health programmes should:

- Not attempt to coerce adults to lead healthy lives.

- Minimise the use of measures that are implemented without consulting people (either individually or using democratic procedures).
- Minimise measures that are very intrusive or conflict with important aspects of personal life, such as privacy.

Consent

Individual consent is not always relevant or appropriate when considering public health measures. For example, individual consent might be unnecessary if the measure is not very intrusive or if it prevents significant harm to others. Furthermore, in some situations it may be more appropriate to obtain approval from the population as a whole (through democratic decision-making procedures), in particular where there is only a limited degree of interference with individuals' liberty and no substantial health risks (Nuffield Council on Bioethics, 2007)

Applying the stewardship model

The components of the stewardship model are not listed in any order of priority, and the different elements could come into conflict – for example, the elements of protecting children and minimising intrusion into private life. There is no set rule for resolving these conflicts. However, the overall aim should be to achieve the desired health outcomes while minimising restrictions on people's freedom (Nuffield Council on Bioethics, 2007).

The National Institute for Health and Care Excellence (NICE) has adopted the Council's stewardship model for public health 'as a reference point for guiding decisions about what types of intervention may be justified' (Nuffield Council on Bioethics, 2010).

Opportunity and choice versus coercion

Figure 6.6.1 An example of a 'nudge'. Source: National Health Service. Licensed under Open Government Licence v3.0. http://www.nationalarchives.gov.uk/doc/open-government-licence/version/3/.

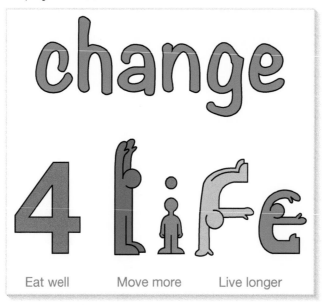

Eat well   Move more   Live longer

Box 6.6.1 Examples of intervention techniques. Source: Data from Local Government Association (2013).

Smacks

- Eliminating choice – banning goods or services such as the restriction on smoking in public places.

Hugs

- Financial incentives – vouchers in exchange for healthy behaviour.

Nudges

- Provision of information – calorie counts on menus.
- Changes to environment – designing buildings with fewer lifts.
- Changes to default – making salad the default side option instead of chips.
- Use of norms – providing information about what others are doing.

Shoves

- Financial disincentives – taxation on cigarettes.
- Restricting choice – banning takeaways from setting up close to schools.

Public Health and Health Promotion for Nurses at a Glance, First Edition. Karen Wild and Maureen McGrath.
© 2019 John Wiley & Sons Ltd. Published 2019 by John Wiley & Sons Ltd.

The UK government is compelled to persuade people to adopt more healthy lifestyles and it does this in three key ways:
- Firstly by setting standards for national health by, for example, clean air and water legislation.
- Secondly by curtailing individual freedom by, for example, banning smoking in public spaces, or by compulsory wearing of helmets whist driving or being a passenger on a motorcycle.
- The third way is to control and legislate about how health messages can be incorporated into commercial products through advertising and labelling. This has been a focus of recent coalitions who have introduced a 'sugar tax' on fizzy drinks in the UK.

Whilst direct instruction or overt enforcement of healthier behaviour can be effective, a more ethically sound approach to better support the principle of autonomy has come into vogue – the so-called 'nudge' theory.

Nudging

Nudge theory can be described as a policy approach to the science of human behaviour. The theory suggests that positive reinforcement of behaviours, coupled with hints and suggestions, can (subconsciously) influence an individual's drive, incentive, cooperation and choice processes in relation to health. Nudge-type interventions that steer people in certain directions while maintaining their freedom of choice result in unconscious behaviours and decisions about health. Being unaware that our thoughts, behaviours and attitudes to health are being influenced by an external force is a key component of the success of nudging.

Poor diet and obesity are making Britain ill and this comes with a price. The burden this places on the NHS is estimated at £12.5 billion a year in avoidable care costs, much bigger than that from smoking, and it is growing. Ethicists argue that state intervention is an act of paternal libertarianism and as such, paternalistic acts of guiding and nudging are justified. In this case examples such as having salad as a default option at the school canteen instead of chips, and placing more emphasis on lower fat options such as pasta and rice dishes as opposed to fried food, can be morally justified. The 'change 4 life' campaign (Figure 6.6.1) is another example.

Other interventions to influence behaviour

Box 6.6.1 highlights a more comprehensive range of interventions that can influence behaviour.
- Direct incentives, such as vouchers in return for healthy behaviour, are being labelled **'hugs'**. Examples include prescriptions for gym membership, and vouchers for slimming club membership. The expectation is that there will be a degree of reciprocity and opportunity for the individual and health professional to engage in health promotion activities.
- More extreme examples that impose tougher restrictions on choice have been labelled **'shoves'**. Restrictions such as the removal of perceived unhealthy options could be applied here. The school canteen options in this example would simply remove the chips and fried food selection from the menu, thereby **shoving** the pupils to choose healthier options. Some councils have adopted a restriction on the percentage of food outlets within a geographical area.
- **Smacks** impose the harshest restrictions, banning activities and compelling individuals to behave in a predetermined manner.

Ethical argument

Nudge theory and its ethical acceptance has raised doubt and uncertainty focusing on its efficacy as a standard approach to influence healthy behaviour. Claims that nudging and allied interventions can control people without them knowing it sits uneasily with health-care professionals. However, the counter argument presents the other side of nudging that exists to encourage unhealthy behaviours used by huge organisations in marketing campaigns. Theorists talk about the obesogenic environment in which we live – high streets and public places such as shopping centres and cinemas are dominated by shops selling fried chicken, burgers, sugary drinks, pasties and sweets. A range of sensory prompts are regularly used by supermarkets and the food industry to encourage shoppers to buy their products; however, this is considered ethically wrong as it could be argued behavioural change is a form of covert coercion.

Individual versus collective interests in public health strategies

Figure 6.7.1 Proportional contributions of major health determinants to premature deaths in the UK. Source: Public Health England, 2016. Licensed under Open Government Licence v3.0. http://www.nationalarchives.gov.uk/doc/open- government-licence/version/3/.

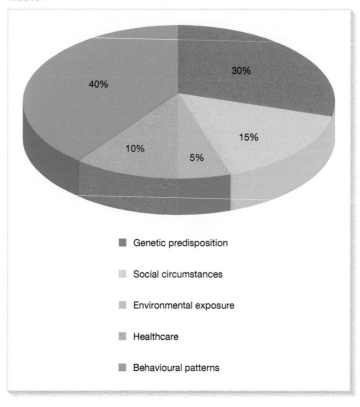

■ Genetic predisposition

■ Social circumstances

■ Environmental exposure

■ Healthcare

■ Behavioural patterns

Public Health and Health Promotion for Nurses at a Glance, First Edition. Karen Wild and Maureen McGrath.
© 2019 John Wiley & Sons Ltd. Published 2019 by John Wiley & Sons Ltd.

The health and wellbeing of individuals and populations across all age groups is influenced by a range of factors both within and outside the individual's control (see Chapter 3 in Unit 1). The Dahlgren and Whitehead (1991) model provides a framework within its layers to analyse the contribution of each of the layers to health. This framework has helped researchers in public health to construct a range of ideas about the origin of negative health determinants, for example from genetic pre-dispositions, a person's social circumstances, environmental exposures, individual behaviour or shortfalls in medical care. Figure 6.7.1 highlights the proportional contribution to premature death from major health determinants in the UK in 2016. On a regular basis in health care, nurses see the consequences of poor health arising from personal lifestyle choices that collectively present major public health challenges: poor diet, smoking and addictions to name a few.

In the past, major population-wide public health interventions dramatically changed individual experiences of health in this country. Traditional public health concerns focused on eradicating communicable diseases and improving health and safety. Contemporary interventions now focus on lifestyle choices and the long-term consequences to individual health and the burden that this places on public health provision. In its 2010 white paper, Healthy Lives, Healthy People (Department of Health, 2010), the then coalition government championed the idea of individual choice and personal responsibility as a way forward in promoting healthy lifestyles. Linking the two ideas of freedom and responsibility can present difficult ethical problems. The principle of autonomy or choice is not confined to the individual; there are often environmental or social pressures that impact upon individual choice, for example:

- The availability of cheap alcohol.
- Marketing of food high in sugar, fat or salt to children.
- A move to more sedentary work patterns.
- Availability of transport.

Autonomy can only be meaningful if individuals have the facility to influence their lives. From an ethical standpoint, as a correlative to autonomy, the state has an obligation to provide conditions where individual choices can thrive.

Individual choices and inequality

Our health choices are determined by a wealth of factors; they are often influenced by our upbringing and environment, and are subject to the distribution of life chances, good and not so good. As such, choices around health behaviour become more difficult. People in the lower social gradients find it more difficult to make healthy choices and to take advantage of health promotion interventions. This basic fact of life can be considered an ethical justification for state intervention in public health.

State intervention and health

Public Health England (PHE) (2016) has set out its plan to address health interventions:

- Support people to make healthy choices, through the refreshed Change4Life programme, and maximise the impact on the public's health of the age 40–60 healthy behaviours campaign ('One You') to inspire and support positive behaviour change.
- Create a suite of digital content, apps and tools that support families and individuals to make changes (an example is the Sugar Smart app) and ensure that nurses engage effectively with people through social channels as well as local and national media and other settings.
- Continue the Act Fast campaign that highlights stroke signs.
- Continue the Be Clear on Cancer campaign that gets more people to recognise symptoms that might indicate cancer, and to see their GP earlier.
- Deliver the Information Service for Parents and the Start4Life campaign, addressing maternal and early years health.
- Continue the Rise Above and Frank digital programmes to address prevention of uptake of exploratory behaviours in teens.
- Recommission a new national HIV home testing sampling service to over 50 000 individuals to support NHS England and local government in improving prevention through targeted information and resources to enable people to make safer and sustainable sexual health choices.
- Raise awareness of the risk factors of dementia and the best steps to mitigate them.
- Test a public awareness approach to antimicrobial resistance.

8 Individual versus collective interests in public health. Example 1 – Alcohol

Figure 6.8.1 Alcohol is the third leading risk factor for death and disability after smoking and obesity. Source: National Health Service. Licensed under Open Government Licence v3.0. http://www.nationalarchives.gov.uk/doc/open-government-licence/version/3/.

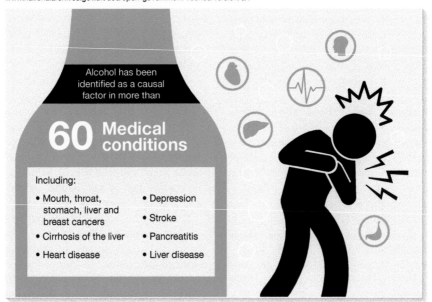

Figure 6.8.2 The 'Know Your Limits' campaign. Source: Drinkaware. Reproduced with permission of Drinkaware.

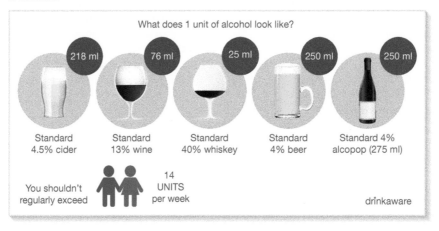

Alcohol consumption

In Great Britain in 2014, there were 28.9 million people who reported that they drank alcohol in the week before being interviewed for the Opinions and Lifestyle Survey. This equates to 58% of the population (ONS, 2016). The National Institute for Health and Care Excellence (NICE, 2011) defines harmful drinking as 'a pattern of alcohol consumption that causes health problems, including psychological problems such as depression, alcohol-related accidents or physical illness such as acute pancreatitis'. The Chief Medical Officer (CMO) has published alcohol guidelines that state that drinking any level of alcohol regularly carries a health risk for everyone. Men and women should limit their intake to no more than 14 units a week to keep the risk of illness like cancer and liver disease low. An analysis of 67 risk factors and risk factor clusters for death and disability found that alcohol is the third leading risk factor for death and disability after smoking and obesity (Figure 6.8.1).

The Licensing Act 2003 came into force in 2005 and fundamentally changed the basis on which venues in England are licensed to sell alcohol. It made it possible for venues to open at all hours of the day (if they applied and paid for the appropriate licence). This has commonly been understood as a 'liberalisation' of licensing in the UK. This liberal rhetoric has also been adopted by the government, which acknowledges the role that alcohol has in the long-standing tradition of British culture and reinforces the liberal stance that how, when and how much people drink is down to individual choice.

Individual choice

Personal autonomy is an important value in our society, meaning that individuals should have the freedom to determine the course of their own lives without unnecessary restrictions. Alcohol consumption is viewed by many as pleasurable and harmless, and will cite the 'French paradox' to support the notion that alcohol can even have health benefits. The intervention ladder shows how autonomy can be constrained and supported.

The intervention ladder

Applying the different levels of the intervention ladder might create varied state-led interventions.

1 **Eliminate choice** – introduce a total ban on sale or even the use of alcohol.

2 **Restrict choice** – introduce licensing laws that only allow alcohol to be sold at restricted times in controlled outlets. Restrictions on advertising might also come here.

3 **Guide choice through disincentives** – increase taxes on alcoholic drinks, and inhibit cheap offers that encourage excessive drinking.

4 **Guide choices through incentives** – make low-alcohol/non-alcoholic drinks cheaper.

5 **Guide choices through changing payment policy** – restaurants and bars always provide free water.

6 **Enable choice** – ensure that desirable non-alcoholic drinks are always available, such as pubs serving coffee.

7 **Provide information** – the 'know your units' labelling (Figure 6.8.2).

8 **Do nothing**.

The impact of alcohol misuse on children and families

From an ethical standpoint, consequentialists may invoke the principle of non-malifice as a reason to exercise paternalism where there is excessive alcohol consumption. Public Health England (2016) presents the following evidence:

• Alcohol misuse impacts not just on the drinker but also those around them. Children affected by parental alcohol misuse are more likely to have physical, psychological and behavioural problems.

• Parental alcohol misuse is strongly correlated with family conflict and with domestic violence and abuse. This poses a risk to children of immediate significant harm and of longer-term negative consequences.

• Alcohol plays a part in 25–33% of known cases of child abuse.

• In a study of four London boroughs, almost two-thirds of all children subject to care proceedings had parents who misused substances including alcohol.

• In a study of young offending cases where the young person was also misusing alcohol, 78% had a history of parental alcohol abuse or domestic abuse within the family (Public Health England, 2016)

• Alcohol misuse also affects carers and adult family members. The Care Act 2014 recognises this and recommends an assessment of their own needs (Public Health England, 2016).

9 Individual versus collective interests in public health. Example 2 – People with learning disabilities

Figure 6.9.1 Health risks associated with inequalities for children with learning disabilities. Source: Public Health England (2015). Licensed under Open Government Licence v3.0. http://www.nationalarchives.gov.uk/doc/open-government-licence/version/3/.

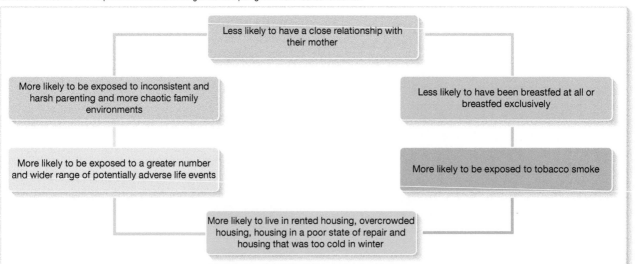

Table 6.9.1 Some of the formal inquiries into learning disabilities health care.

Inquiry	Aims/outcomes
Valuing People (Department of Health) – 2001	Aims to challenge established practice to improve services. This was the first White Paper on learning disability for 30 years (DH, 2001)
Treat Me Right (Mencap) – 2004	Exposed inequalities in health care for people with learning disabilities
Disability Rights Commission Report – 2006	Exposed that little or nothing had been done by the government to adhere to the recommendations of Mencap's 'Treat Me Right' report
Death by Indifference (Mencap) – 2007	Highlighted circumstances surrounding the deaths of six adults with learning disabilities while they were in the care of the NHS, suggesting that people with learning disabilities, their families and carers were facing institutional discrimination in health-care services (Mencap, 2007)
Healthcare for All – 2008	The report of the 'Michael Inquiry' set up to learn lessons from the six cases highlighted in the Mencap report ('Death by Indifference'). It reported evidence of 'a significant level of avoidable suffering and a high likelihood that there are deaths occurring which could be avoided'
High Quality Care for All – 2008	Lord Darzi sets out a 10-year plan to provide the highest quality of care, including improvements to those patients with disabilities
Valuing People Now – 2009	Sets targets to change the approach to learning disability services. The strategy covers all areas of a person's life
The Autism Act – 2009	Building on the success of the 'I Exist Campaign', the Act made two key provisions: that the government produce an adult autism strategy by 1 April 2010 and that the Secretary of State for Health issues, by 31 December 2010, statutory guidance for local authorities and local health bodies on supporting the needs of adults with autism
Death by Indifference: 74 Deaths and Counting – 2012	Highlights further unnecessary deaths of people with a learning disability and notes lack of compliance with the Equality Act (2010) and the failure to make 'reasonable adjustments' and comply with the Mental Capacity Act, 2005
Six Lives Progress Report on Healthcare for People with Learning Disabilities – 2013	The regulatory system through the Care Quality Commission (CQC), Monitor and professional regulation works to ensure that people with learning disabilities are protected when using health and care services
Confidential Inquiry into Premature Deaths of People with Learning Disabilities (CIPOLD) – 2013	The Confidential Inquiry into the Deaths of People with Learning disabilities (CIPOLD) was tasked with investigating the avoidable or premature deaths of people with learning disabilities through a series of retrospective reviews of deaths. The aim was to review the patterns of care that people received in the period leading up to their deaths, to identify errors or omissions contributing to those deaths, to illustrate evidence of good practice, and to provide improved evidence on avoiding premature death

Public Health and Health Promotion for Nurses at a Glance, First Edition. Karen Wild and Maureen McGrath.
© 2019 John Wiley & Sons Ltd. Published 2019 by John Wiley & Sons Ltd.

Figure 6.9.2 Headline findings from the Learning Disabilities Health and Care Project. Source: Public Health England (2016). Licensed under Open Government Licence v3.0. http://www.nationalarchives.gov.uk/doc/open-government-licence/version/3/.

Weight	Being underweight was 1.8 times as common for people with learning disabilities as for others; being obese was 1.3 times as common. By contrast people with learning disabilities were less likely to be a healthy weight or a little overweight but without reaching the obesity threshold
Common long-term health conditions	People with learning disabilities were between 1.5 and 2 times as likely to have a diagnosis of Asthma Chronic kidney disease Diabetes (Type 1 and non-type 1) Heart failure Stroke or transient ischaemic attack People with learning disabilities were less likely to have a diagnosis of coronary heart disease or chronic obstructive pulmonary disease People with learning disabilities were more than 8 times as likely to have a diagnosis of a severe mental illness. This is more than research suggests is likely Diagnosis of difficulty swallowing (dysphagia) was only half as common as research suggests likely Diabetes management in people with learning disability seemed as effective in producing good long-term blood sugar control as in diabetics without learning disabilities
Health checks	43% of people with learning disabilities had a record of a learning disabilities health check in the previous year
Influenza immunisations	41% had an influenza immunisation in the previous winter
Cancer screening	Cervical cancer screening coverage for women with learning disabilities was only 40% of the rate for people without Breast cancer screening coverage for women with learning disabilities was 80% of the rate for people without Colorectal cancer screening coverage for people with learning disabilities was 90% of the rate for people without
Palliative care	Adjusting for age, people with learning disabilities were 3.3 times as likely to be receiving terminal palliative care
Mortality	Death rates were higher for people with learning disabilities. Allowing for their age profile, there were 3.3 times the expected number of deaths among women with learning disabilities, and 2.7 times the expected number among men. Life expectancy at birth for women was reduced by 18 years and for men by 14 years

Learning disabilities

The learning disability population has poorer health than the general population and is more likely to experience mental illness, epilepsy, physical disability and sensory impairments, as well as chronic health problems. In addition to this, people with learning disabilities experience a shorter life expectancy than people in the mainstream population. However, they are less likely to access health care in a way that the rest of us take for granted. Mencap (2007, p.18) states that 'it is Mencap's belief that there is institutional discrimination within the NHS against people with a learning disability leading to neglect and, as we have shown, to premature death.' These health inequalities have been highlighted in a number of formal inquiries (Table 6.9.1).

A range of barriers to accessing health care and other services have been identified; these include:

- Scarcity of appropriate services.
- Physical and informational barriers to access.
- Unhelpful, inexperienced or discriminatory health-care staff.
- Increasingly stringent eligibility criteria for accessing social care services.
- Failure of health-care providers to make 'reasonable adjustments' in light of the literacy and communication difficulties experienced by many people with learning disabilities.
- 'Diagnostic overshadowing' (e.g. symptoms of physical ill health being mistakenly attributed to either a mental health/behavioural problem or regarded as being inherent in the person's learning disabilities) (Peate and Wild, 2017).

In its report, 'Shaping the Future, A Vision for Learning Disabilities Nursing', the UK Learning Disability Consultant Nurse Network (2006) stated that:

Learning disability nurses must ensure that they are fully aware of the developing evidence base regarding the health needs of, and disparities experienced by, people with learning disabilities. They must utilise this evidence to challenge inequalities and inequities in health and challenge the barriers to good health.

Public Health England (2015) identified health inequalities experienced by children with learning disabilities. Using evidence and scientific knowledge, a range of determinants that contribute to those inequalities were identified. Figure 6.9.1 highlights the determinants and shows the kinds of risks that such children can be exposed to.

Public health needs of people with learning difficulties

Annual learning disability health checks were introduced in 2008–9. They are a key recommended 'reasonable adjustment' in providing primary care for this group who may benefit from early screening and intervention, and who might not be aware that their GP could help with emerging physical problems. They have been shown to identify many previously unsuspected, common, distressing and potentially treatable conditions. Table 6.9.2 highlights the headline findings from the Learning Disabilities Health and Care Project (Public Health England, 2016). The findings make a comparison between the health of people with learning disabilities and those who don't have a learning disability.

Consent and best interests

Seen as a core aspect of the nurse's role, consent is important and is underpinned in 'The Code' (NMC, 2015) when it asks nurses to listen to people and respond to their preferences and concerns. When applied within the field of learning disabilities, consent fulfils important tasks. It establishes and safeguards the autonomy of the individual and is a necessary and legal component of health care within the UK. Gaining consent from people with learning disabilities can be complex and challenging. Making valued decisions about an individual's capacity to provide consent requires an understanding of what constitutes a person's best interests, and an understanding of how to assess cognitive impairment and a person's ability to understand the consequences of health-related interventions. For a person's consent to be valid, the person must be:

- Capable of taking that particular decision ('competent').
- Acting voluntarily (not under pressure or duress from anyone).
- Provided with enough information to enable them to make the decision (DH, 2001).

10 Ethical issues in engaging people in conversations about health: an overview

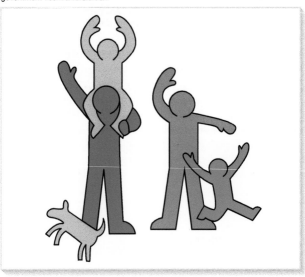

Figure 6.10.1   Change 4 Life. Source: National Health Service. Licensed under Open Government Licence v3.0. http://www.nationalarchives.gov.uk/doc/open-government-licence/version/3/.

Box 6.10.1   'The Code'. Source: NMC (2015).

Listen to people and respond to their preferences and concerns. To achieve this, you must:

2.1 Work in partnership with people to make sure you deliver care effectively.

2.2 Recognise and respect the contribution that people can make to their own health and wellbeing.

2.3 Encourage and empower people to share decisions about their treatment and care.

2.4 Respect the level to which people receiving care want to be involved in decisions about their own health, wellbeing and care.

2.5 Respect, support and document a person's right to accept or refuse care and treatment, and

2.6 Recognise when people are anxious or in distress and respond compassionately and politely.

Introduction

As health promoters, nurses are ideally placed to offer information, advice and support and to screen and encourage people to adopt healthy behaviours. A variety of chapters within this text have highlighted the approaches that nurses can engage in when communicating with groups and individuals to achieve such aims. The process of health promotion makes it necessary for nurses to influence individual's beliefs, views, choices, behaviour, relationships and lifestyles. It is this method of health promotion that raises the question of ethical and moral approaches, where influence and persuasion are the norm.

Types of ethical concerns

As nurses, we are in a unique position. People who are in our care may not consider an infringement on their privacy as an ethical concern. Nurses may interpret a patient's cooperation as a signal and agreement of trust and consent. An example might be the assumption that an individual is happy to have antiembolic stockings applied by the nurse prior to surgery. It is imperative that the individual gives consent before any treatment, care or examination. If an individual refuses intervention, but it still goes ahead, then this is a civil or criminal wrong, so-called 'trespass against the person', and nurses could see themselves falling foul of assault and battery, and be called to account by the Nursing and Midwifery Council (NMC). Harm in this situation can result in an accusation of negligence on the part of the nurse.

For consent to be valid, there are three key principles that have to be satisfied:

1 Consent is **informed**
2 The individual is **competent**
3 Consent is **voluntary**.

Box 6.10.1 identifies the parts of 'The Code' (NMC, 2015) that make this explicit.

Of course the obligations to avoid harm (maleficence) and do good (non-maleficence) are of prime importance; however, interventions can in the short or long term fail to meet these obligations. Health promotion activities can cause harm, directly or indirectly, in a physical, social, psychological or cultural manner. Examples might include anxiety and social stigma, or the lack of support services to adequately manage ongoing health promotion.

However, health promotion activities that are educational or discreet, or are carried out by the media, or government campaigns (such as Public health England's 'Change 4 Life'

campaign – Figure 6.10.1) can be interpreted as holding public approval. Such interventions focus on the teleological or utilitarian approach to ethics, that which represents the greatest benefit to people or society.

Respecting autonomy supports the right of individuals to make their own decisions and choices with regard to their current and future health. This is acceptable as long as the right to a person's autonomy does not infringe on others' rights or inflicts harm on others. It also brings into question the individual's ability to choose and the obligation on the part of health services and social situations to uphold that choice. An example might be healthy eating: a person might choose healthy options, but within the context of family and culture, those choices might conflict with the choices of others in that situation.

The fair and equitable distribution of resources presents a degree of contention within health promotion. As nurses we strive to understand the determinants of health and the subsequent inequalities that exist in our patient groups. We actively support large-scale health promotion programmes, often government led, to inform our interventions. Paradoxically, large-scale programmes that target aspects of health such as early cancer detection, heart disease, obesity and physical health are more likely to have an impact on the more affluent groups of society.

Caring in the context of nursing implies the obligation to be connected with one's patients and clients. From a professional and values perspective, this includes the obligation to communicate, show compassion, be receptive and responsive to others' needs, be sincere, genuine, and impart a sense of trust in those who are cared for. Health promotion engages the nurse in informing, persuading, facilitating, decision-making and advocating for the individual. Veracity (truth telling) can be a difficult ethical issue when facing the realities of health with patients or clients. Clear and simple information in small doses may be more acceptable to some. The most compelling argument in favour of full disclosure is that patients are then in the best position to make choices (exercise autonomy) about how their treatment will develop. By telling the truth to patients, nurses imply a genuine concern for the person's wellbeing and are demonstrating a link to the principle of beneficence. Autonomy is closely related to dignity and it could be argued that by not telling an individual the truth, their dignity is undermined. It can also be argued that the person's best interests can be affected. Disclosure of information may go a long way to influence the choices that a patient makes in relation to healthy behaviour.

Appendix

Figure 1.8.2 NHS screening timeline. Source: National Health Service. Licensed under Open Government Licence v3.0. http://www.nationalarchives.gov.uk/doc/open-government-licence/version/3/www.screening.nhs.uk/england.

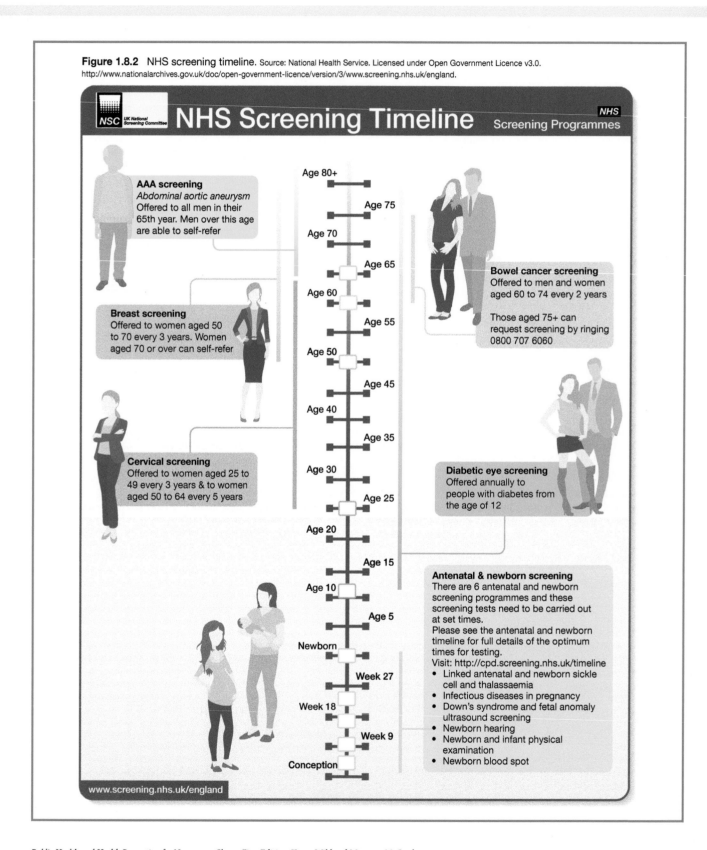

Public Health and Health Promotion for Nurses at a Glance, First Edition. Karen Wild and Maureen McGrath.
© 2019 John Wiley & Sons Ltd. Published 2019 by John Wiley & Sons Ltd.

References

Chapter 1.1: What is public health and why is it relevant to nursing?

Acheson, D. (1988) Public Health in England: The Report of the Committee of Inquiry into the Future Development to the Public Health Function. London: DHSS.

Department of Health (2010) Healthy Lives, Healthy People. London: DH. Available at: https://www.gov.uk/government/uploads/system/uploads/attachment_data/file/216096/dh_127424.pdf (accessed 19 March 2018).

Department of Health (2012) The Public Health Outcomes Framework for England 2013-2016. London: DH. Available at: https://www.gov.uk/government/uploads/system/uploads/attachment_data/file/216159/dh_132362.pdf (accessed 19 March 2018).

Marmot, M. (2010) Fair society, healthy lives: the Marmot Review: strategic review of health inequalities in England post-2010. Available at: http://www.instituteofhealthequity.org/resources-reports/fair-society-healthy-lives-the-marmot-review (accessed 15 may 2018).

Nursing and Midwifery Council (2015) Standards for competence for registered nurses. London: NMC. Available at: http://www.nmc.org.uk/globalassets/sitedocuments/standards/nmc-standards-for-competence-for-registered-nurses.pdf (accessed 19 March 2018).

Wilkinson, R. and Pickett, K. (2010) The Spirit Level. London: Penguin.

Chapter 1.2: Some historical points of public health

Rosen, G. (1993) A History of Public Health. Baltimore: Johns Hopkins University Press. Cited in Costello, J. and Haggart, M. (2003) Public Health and Society. Basingstoke: Palgrave Macmillan.

Chapter 1.3: Determinants of health

Bunker, J.P., Frazier, H.S. and Mosteller, F. (1995) The role of medical care in determining health: Creating an inventory of benefits. In: Amick, B.C. III, Levine, S., Tarlov, A.R. and Chapman Walsh, D. (eds) Society and Health. New York: Oxford University Press, pp. 305–341.

Canadian Institute of Advanced Research, Health Canada, Population and Public Health Branch. AB/NWT 2002, quoted in Kuznetsova, D. (2012) Healthy places: Councils leading on public health. London: New Local Government Network. Available at: http://www.nlgn.org.uk/public/2012/healthy-places-councils-leading-on-public-health/ (accessed 20 March 2018).

Dahlgren, G. and Whitehead, M. (1991) Policies and Strategies to Promote Social Equity in Health. Stockholm: Institute of Futures Studies.

Marmot, M. (2010) Fair society, healthy lives: the Marmot Review: strategic review of health inequalities in England post-2010. Available at: http://www.instituteofhealthequity.org/resources-reports/fair-society-healthy-lives-the-marmot-review (accessed 15 may 2018).

McGinnis, J.M., Williams-Russo, P. and Knickman, J.R. (2002) The case for more active policy attention to health promotion. Health Affairs 21(2), 78–93.

World Health Organization (1988) Making partners: intersectoral action for health: proceedings and outcome of a joint working group on intersectoral action for health, Utrecht, The Netherlands, 30 November–2 December 1988. WHO Regional Office for Europe.

Chapter 1.4: Health improvement and the role of the nurse

Ball, J.E., Murrells, T., Rafferty, A.M., Morrow, E. and Griffiths, P. (2013) 'Care left undone' during nursing shifts: associations with workload and perceived quality of care. BMJ Quality and Safety online; doi:10.1136/bmjqs-2012-001767.

Department of Health (2012) The Public Health Outcomes Framework for England, 2013-2016. London: DH. Available at: https://www.gov.uk/government/uploads/system/uploads/attachment_data/file/216159/dh_132362.pdf (accessed 20 March 2018).

Department of Health (2012) The NHS's role in the public's health. A report from the NHS Future Forum. DH, London.

Department of Health and Public Health England (2013) Nursing and midwifery actions at the three levels of public health practice. Improving health and wellbeing at individual, community and population levels. London: DH. Available at: https://www.gov.uk/government/uploads/system/uploads/attachment_data/file/208814/3_Levels.pdf (accessed 20 March 2018).

Ford, S. (2014) Exclusive survey: Nurses underpaid, overworked and undervalued. Nursing Times 7 May 2014.

Miller, W.R. and Rollnick, S. (2002) Motivational Interviewing: Preparing People to Change Addictive Behavior, 2nd edn. New York: Guilford Press.

National Obesity Observatory (2011) Brief Interventions for Weight Management. Available at: https://www.hse.ie/eng/health/child/healthyeating/weightmanagement.pdf (accessed 15 May 2018).

NHS Commissioning Board and Department of Health (2012) Compassion in Practice. London: NHS Commissioning Board. Available at: http://www.england.nhs.uk/wp-content/uploads/2012/12/compassion-in-practice.pdf (accessed 20 March 2018).

NHS England et al. (2014) Five Year Forward View. London: NHS England. Available at: http://www.england.nhs.uk/wp-content/uploads/2014/10/5yfv-web.pdf (accessed 20 March 2018).

NICE (National Institute for Health & Care Excellence) (2006) Smoking: Brief Interventions and Referrals. Manchester: NICE. Available at: https://www.nice.org.uk/guidance/ph1 (accessed 15 May 2018).

NICE (National Institute for Health & Care Excellence) (2014) Obesity: identification, assessment and management. Available at: https://www.nice.org.uk/guidance/cg189/chapter/1-recommendations (accessed 20 March 2018).

Public Health and Health Promotion for Nurses at a Glance, First Edition. Karen Wild and Maureen McGrath.
© 2019 John Wiley & Sons Ltd. Published 2019 by John Wiley & Sons Ltd.

Royal College of Nursing (2012) Going upstream. Nursing's contribution to public health. Available at: https://mafiadoc .com/going-upstream-nursings-contribution-to-public-health-pdf-rcn_59decea11723ddca22f3bce5.html (accessed 28 March 2018).

World Health Organization (2010) Brief Intervention – The ASSIST-linked brief intervention for hazardous and harmful substance use. Manual for use in primary care. Geneva: WHO. Available at: http://whqlibdoc.who.int/publications/2010/9789241599399_eng .pdf?ua=1 (accessed 20 March 2018).

Chapter 1.5: What people think about public health

BMA (2016) Public Perceptions of the NHS. Britain Thinks, Survey Results. London: British Medical Association.

Department of Health (2012) Liberating the NHS. No Decision About Me Without Me. London: DH.

Department of Health (2013) Public Perceptions of the NHS and Social Care Survey. Winter 2013 Waves. London: DH.

Office for National Statistics (2016) Number of deaths and age standardised rate (per 100,000 population) for Dementia and Alzheimer's deaths (combined), based on deaths registered in England and Wales 2004 to 2014. London: ONS. Available at: https://www.ons.gov.uk/peoplepopulationandcommunity/ birthsdeathsandmarriages/deaths/adhocs/006324numberof deathsandagestandardisedrateper100000populationfor dementiaandalzheimersdeathscombinedbasedondeaths registeredinenglandwales2004to2014 (accessed 20 March 2018).

PHE (2014) Public Awareness and Opinions Survey. Public Health England.

Chapter 1.6: How public health is measured: epidemiology

ONS (Office for National Statistics) (2011) 2011 Census. Available at: http://www.ons.gov.uk/census/2011census (accessed November 2016).

ONS (Office for National Statistics) (2015) Deaths registered in England and Wales 2015. Available at: https://www.ons.gov.uk/ peoplepopulationandcommunity/birthsdeathsandmarriages/ deaths/bulletins/deathsregistrationsummarytables/2015#main-points (accessed 22 March 2018).

ONS (Office for National Statistics) (2016) Life Expectancy at Birth and at Age 65 by Local Areas in England and Wales: 2012 to 2014. Available at: https://www.ons.gov.uk/ peoplepopulationandcommunity/birthsdeathsandmarriages/ lifeexpectancies/bulletins/lifeexpectancyatbirthandatage65by localareasinenglandandwales/2015-11-04 (accessed 22 March 2018).

Chapter 1.7: Public health outcomes and the role of the nurse

Davies, S.C., Winpenny, E., Ball, S., Fowler, T., Rubin, J. and Nolte, E. (2014) For Debate: a new wave in public health improvement. *The Lancet* 384:1889–1895.

Department of Health (2012) The Public Health Outcomes Framework for England, 2013-2016. London: DH. Available at: https://www.gov.uk/government/uploads/system/uploads/ attachment_data/file/216159/dh_132362.pdf (accessed 22 March 2018).

Department of Health & Public Health England (2014) A Framework for Personalised Care and Population Health for Nurses, Midwives, Health Visitors and Allied Health Professionals. Available at: https://www.gov.uk/government/ uploads/system/uploads/attachment_data/file/377450/ Framework_for_personalised_care_and_population_health_ for_nurses.pdf (accessed 22 March 2018).

NMC (Nursing and Midwifery Council) (2015) Standards for competence for registered nurses. Available at: http://www.nmc.org.uk/globalassets/sitedocuments/standards/ nmc-standards-for-competence-for-registered-nurses.pdf (accessed 22 March 2018).

Chapter 1.9: Health surveillance

Dahlgren, G. and Whitehead, M. (1991) *Policies and Strategies to Promote Social Equity in Health*. Stockholm: Institute of Futures Studies.

Wills, J. (2014) *Fundamentals of Health Promotion for Nurses*, 2nd edn. Chichester: Wiley-Blackwell.

World Health Organization (2016) Public health surveillance. Available at: http://www.who.int/topics/public_health_ surveillance/en/ (accessed November 2016).

Chapter 1.10: Inequalities in health

BBC News (2013) Huge survey reveals seven social classes in UK. Available at: http://www.bbc.co.uk/news/uk-22007058 (accessed 24 May 2018).

Marmot, M. (1997) Inequality, deprivation and alcohol use. *Addiction* 92(3 Suppl. 1), 13–20.

Marmot, M. (2010) Fair society, healthy lives: the Marmot Review: strategic review of health inequalities in England post-2010. Available at: http://www.instituteofhealthequity.org/ resourcesreports/fair-society-healthy-lives-the-marmot-review (accessed 24th June 2018).

Marsh, A., Gordon, D., Heslop, P. and Pantazis, C. (2010) Housing deprivation and health: A longitudinal analysis. *Housing Studies* 15(3), 411–428.

Chapter 1.11: Investigations into inequalities in health: reports and reviews

Acheson, D. (1998) *Independent Inquiry Into Inequalities in Health*. London: HMSO, Department of Health.

DHSS (1980) *Inequalities in Health (The Black Report)*. London: DHSS.

Marmot, M. (2010) *Fair Society Healthy Lives*. The Marmot Review. London: Institute of Health Equity.

Chapter 1.12: The relationship between public health and competency standards for registered nurses

NHS England (2016) Leading Change, Adding Value: a framework for nursing, midwifery and care staff. NHS England. Available at: https://www.england.nhs.uk/wp-content/uploads/2016/05/ nursing-framework.pdf (accessed 22 March 2018).

NMC (Nursing and Midwifery Council) (2010) Standards for pre-registration nursing education. London: NMC. Available at: http://www.nmc.org.uk/globalassets/sitedocuments/ nmc-publications/standards-for-pre-registration-nursing-education-16082010.pdf (accessed 22 March 2018).

NMC (Nursing and Midwifery Council) (2014) Standards for competence for registered nurses. Available at: http://www.nmc. org.uk/globalassets/sitedocuments/standards/nmc-standards-for-competence-for-registered-nurses.pdf (accessed 22 March 2018).

The Mid Staffordshire NHS Foundation Trust Public Inquiry (2013) Report of the Mid Staffordshire NHS Foundation Trust Public Inquiry: Executive summary (Chair: R. Francis).

London: Stationery Office. Available at: http://webarchive.nationalarchives.gov.uk/20150407084003/http://www.midstaffspublicinquiry.com/sites/default/files/report/Executive%20summary.pdf (accessed 22 March 2018).

Chapter 2.1: Health promotion

Department of Health and Public Health England (2014) A Framework for Personalised Care and Population Health for Nurses, Midwives, Health Visitors and Allied Health Professionals. Available at: https://www.gov.uk/government/uploads/system/uploads/attachment_data/file/377450/Framework_for_personalised_care_and_population_health_for_nurses.pdf (accessed 23 March 2018).

NHS England (2016) Leading Change Adding Value. A framework for nursing, midwifery and care staff. Available at: https://www.england.nhs.uk/wp-content/uploads/2016/05/nursing-framework.pdf (accessed 23 March 2018).

Public Health England (2016) All Our Health: about the framework. Available at: https://www.gov.uk/government/publications/all-our-health-about-the-framework/all-our-health-about-the-framework (accessed 23 March 2018).

World Health Organization (1986) The Ottawa Charter for Health Promotion. First International Conference on Health Promotion, Ottawa. Available at: http://www.who.int/healthpromotion/conferences/previous/ottawa/en/ (accessed 24 May 2018).

World Health Organization (2016) 9th Global Conference on Health Promotion – resources. Available at: http://www.who.int/healthpromotion/conferences/9gchp/resources/en/ (accessed 23 March 2018).

Chapter 2.2: Aspects of health promotion

Beattie, A. (1991) Knowledge and control in health promotion. In: Calnan, M., Gabe, J. and Bury, M. (eds) *The Sociology of the Health Service*. London: Routledge, pp. 162–202.

GOV.UK (2012 updated 2015) Health Visiting Attributes. Available at: https://assets.publishing.service.gov.uk/government/uploads/system/uploads/attachment_data/file/216454/dh_133017.pdf (accessed 24 May 2018).

Green, J. and Tones, K. (2010) *Health Promotion Planning and Strategies*. London: Sage.

McIlfatrick, S, Keeney, S., Mckenna, S.H. and McIlwee, G. (2013) Exploring the actual and potential role of the primary care nurse in the prevention of cancer: A mixed methods study. *European Journal of Cancer Care* 23(3): 1–12.

Nuffield Council on Bioethics (2007) Public health: ethical issues. London: Nuffield Council on Bioethics. Available at: http://nuffieldbioethics.org/project/public-health (accessed 24 May 2018).

Tannahill, A. (2009) Health Promotion: The Tannahill model revisited. *Public Health* 123: 396–399.

Thomas, S. and Stewart, J. (2004) Health promotion in context. *Environmental Health Journal* December, pp. 382–384.

Tones, K. and Tilford, S. (1994) *Health Education, Effectiveness, Efficiency and Equity*. London: Chapman & Hall.

Chapter 2.3: Primary and secondary prevention of ill health and health education 1. Cardiovascular disease in men

Marmot, M., Oldfield, Z., Clemens, S., Blake, M., Phelps, A., Nazroo, J., et al. (2017) English Longitudinal Study of Ageing: Waves 0–7, 1998–2015 [data collection], 27th edn. UK Data Service, SN: 5050. Available at: https://discover.ukdataservice.ac.uk/catalogue/?sn=5050 (accessed 23 March 2018).

National Institute for Health and Care Excellence (2016) Cardiovascular disease: risk assessment and reduction, including lipid modification. Available at: https://www.nice.org.uk/guidance/cg181 (accessed 23 March 2018).

Office for National Statistics (2017) What are the top causes of death by age and gender. Available at: http://visual.ons.gov.uk/what-are-the-top-causes-of-death-by-age-a (accessed 23 March 2018).

Chapter 2.4: Primary and secondary prevention of ill health and health education 2. Children's dental health

Public Health England (2013) National Dental Epidemiology Programme for England: oral health survey of five-year-old children 2012. A report on the prevalence and severity of dental decay. Available at: http://www.nwph.net/dentalhealth/Oral%20Health%205yr%20old%20children%202012%20final%20report%20gateway%20approved.pdf (accessed 26 march 2018).

Chapter 2.5: Primary and secondary prevention of ill health and health education 3. Self-harm

Mind (2017a) What is self-harm? Available at: http://www.mind.org.uk/information-support/types-of-mental-health-problems/self-harm/#.WNvOp4WcHcs (accessed 26 March 2018).

Mind (2017b) Self-harm. How can I help myself now? Available at: http://www.mind.org.uk/information-support/types-of-mental-health-problems/self-harm/helping-yourself-now/#.WNvPO4WcHcs (accessed 26 March 2018).

Mind (2017c) Self-harm. Distracting yourself from the urge to self-harm. Available at: http://www.mind.org.uk/information-support/types-of-mental-health-problems/self-harm/helping-yourself-now/#distracting (accessed 26 March 2018).

Royal College of Psychiatrists (2017) Self-harm. Available at: https://www.rcpsych.ac.uk/expertadvice/problems/depression/self-harm.aspx (accessed 29 May 2018).

Watson, J. (1997) The theory of human caring: Retrospective and prospective. *Nursing Science Quarterly* 10(1), 49–52.

Chapter 2.6: Primary and secondary prevention of ill health and health education 4. Obesity and people with a learning disability

GOV.UK (2018a) People with learning disabilities. Reasonable adjustments: a legal duty. Available at: https://www.gov.uk/government/publications/reasonable-adjustments-for-people-with-learning-disabilities/reasonable-adjustments-a-legal-duty (accessed 29 May 2018).

GOV.UK (2018b) People with learning disabilities. Making reasonable adjustments. Obesity and weight management. Available at: https://www.gov.uk/government/publications/reasonable-adjustments-for-people-with-learning-disabilities/obesity-and-weight-management (accessed 29 May 2018).

The Caroline Walker Trust (2007) Eating well: children and adults with learning disabilities. Nutritional and practical guidelines. Available at: http://www.cwt.org.uk/wp-content/uploads/2015/02/EWLDGuidelines.pdf (accessed 26 March 2018).

Chapter 2.8: Tertiary prevention of ill health and health education: self-harm; obesity in people with a learning disability

GOV.UK (2018) People with learning disabilities. Making reasonable adjustments. Obesity and weight management.

Available at: https://www.gov.uk/government/publications/
reasonable-adjustments-for-people-with-learning-disabilities/
obesity-and-weight-management (accessed 29 May 2018).

Chapter 3.1: Different experiences of health through the life course

Age UK (2014) Evidence Review Loneliness in Later Life. Available at: https://www.ageuk.org.uk/Documents/EN-GB/For-professionals/Research/Age%20UK%20Evidence%20Review%20on%20Loneliness%20July%202014.pdf?dtrk=true (accessed 26 March 2018).

Department of Health (2011) No Health Without Mental Health. Available at: https://www.gov.uk/government/publications/the-mental-health-strategy-for-england (accessed 26 March 2018).

HM Government (2014) Horizon Scanning Programme. Social attitudes of young people. Available at: https://www.gov.uk/government/uploads/system/uploads/attachment_data/file/389086/Horizon_Scanning_-_Social_Attitudes_of_Young_People_report.pdf (accessed 26 March 2018).

Scriven, A. (2010) *Ewles & Simnett: Promoting Health: A Practical Guide*, 6th edn. Ballièrre Tindall.

Willams, B., Bhaumik, C. and Silk, A. (2012) Lifecourse Tracker Interim Summary Report. GfK NOP Social Research. Available at: https://www.gov.uk/government/uploads/system/uploads/attachment_data/file/214896/lifecourse-final.pdf (accessed 26 March 2018).

World Health Organization (2000) The implications for training of embracing a Life Course approach to health. Available at: http://www.who.int/ageing/publications/lifecourse/alc_lifecourse_training_en.pdf (accessed 26 March 2018).

Chapter 3.2: Long-term conditions: all ages

Department of Health (2012) Long Term Conditions Compendium of Information. Available at: https://www.gov.uk/government/uploads/system/uploads/attachment_data/file/216528/dh_134486.pdf (accessed 27 March 2018).

Department of Health (2013) Children and Young People's Health Outcomes Forum – Report of the Long Term Conditions, Disability and Palliative Care Subgroup. Available at: https://www.gov.uk/government/uploads/system/uploads/attachment_data/file/216856/CYP-Long-Term-Conditions.pdf (accessed 27 March 2018).

NHS England (2017) House of Care – a framework for long term condition care. Available at: https://www.england.nhs.uk/ourwork/ltc-op-eolc/ltc-eolc/house-of-care/ (accessed 27 March 2018).

The Kings Fund (2012) Long-term conditions and mental health. The cost of co-morbidities. Available at: https://www.centreformentalhealth.org.uk/Handlers/Download.ashx?IDMF=5ebc622a-f9cf-48f3-bdfd-a404b616c1fd (accessed 27 March 2018).

Chapter 3.3: Cardiovascular diseases

British Heart Foundation (2018) Cardiovascular disease statistics 2018. Available at: https://www.bhf.org.uk/research/heart-statistics/heart-statistics-publications/cardiovascular-disease-statistics-2018 (accessed 1 June 2018).

PHE (2017) Guidance. Health matters: combating high blood pressure. Public Health England.

Chapter 3.4: Respiratory diseases

British Lung Foundation (2016) Chronic obstructive pulmonary disease (COPD) statistics. Available at: https://statistics.blf.org.uk/copd (accessed 1 June 2018).

ONS (2013) Statistical Bulletin. Deaths registered in England and Wales (series DR), 2012. Available at: http://webarchive.nationalarchives.gov.uk/20160107153522/http://www.ons.gov.uk/ons/dcp171778_331565.pdf (accessed 1 June 2018).

Public Health England (2015) Respiratory disease: applying All Our Health. Available at: https://www.gov.uk/government/publications/respiratory-disease-applying-all-our-health/respiratory-disease-applying-all-our-health (accessed 1 June 2018).

Chapter 3.5: Cancers

Cancer Research UK and UK Health Forum (2016) Tipping the scales. Why preventing obesity makes economic sense. Available at: http://www.cancerresearchuk.org/sites/default/files/tipping_the_scales_-_cruk_full_report11.pdf (accessed 27 March 2018).

Chapter 3.6: Child and adolescent mental health

Children's Commissioner for England (2016) Lightning Review: Children's access to school nurses. Available at: https://www.childrenscommissioner.gov.uk/publication/lightning-review-childrens-access-to-school-nurses-to-improve-wellbeing-and-protect-them-from-harm/ (accessed 27 March 2018).

Korkodilos, M. (2016) Reducing child mortality in London. London: Public Health England. Available at: https://assets.publishing.service.gov.uk/government/uploads/system/uploads/attachment_data/file/551123/Reducing_child_deaths_in_London.pdf (accessed 1 June 2018).

Nuffield Foundation (2013) Social trends and mental health: introducing the main findings. London: Nuffield Foundation.

Chapter 3.7: Depression

American Psychiatric Association (2013) *Diagnostic and Statistical Manual of Mental Disorders*, 5th edn. Arlington, VA: American Psychiatric Publishing.

NICE (2016) Depression in adults: recognition and management. Clinical guideline [CG90]. National Institute for Health and Care Excellence.

ONS (2016) Measuring national well-being: Life in the UK. Office for National Statistics. Available at: https://www.ons.gov.uk/peoplepopulationandcommunity/wellbeing (accessed 27 March 2018).

Chapter 3.8: Dementia

Alzheimer's Society (2014) What is Alzheimer's disease? Fact sheet 401. Available at: https://www.alzheimers.org.uk/download/downloads/id/3379/what_is_alzheimers_disease.pdf (accessed 27 March 2018).

Carers Trust (2016) The triangle of care for dementia. Available at: https://professionals.carers.org/triangle-care-dementia (accessed 27 March 2018).

Chapter 4.1: Why is behaviour change difficult?

Bouton, M.E. (2014) Why behaviour change is difficult to sustain. *Preventive Medicine* 68: 29–36.

Cialdini, R.B. (2007) *Influence. The Psychology of Persuasion*. New York: Harper Collins.

Department of Health and Public Health England (2014) A Framework for Personalised Care and Population Health for Nurses, Midwives, Health Visitors and Allied Health Professionals. Caring for populations across the lifecourse. Available at: https://www.gov.uk/government/uploads/system/uploads/attachment_data/file/377450/Framework_for_personalised_care_and_population_health_for_nurses.pdf (accessed 27 March 2018).

Kelly, M.P. and Barker, M. (2016) Why is changing health related behaviour so difficult? *Public Health* 136: 109–116.

NHS England (2016) Leading Change, Adding Value: a framework for nursing, midwifery and care staff. Available at: https://www.england.nhs.uk/wp-content/uploads/2016/05/nursing-framework.pdf (accessed 27 March 2018).

NHS England (2017) Next steps on the NHS five year forward view. Available at: https://www.england.nhs.uk/wp-content/uploads/2017/03/NEXT-STEPS-ON-THE-NHS-FIVE-YEAR-FORWARD-VIEW.pdf (accessed 29 May 2018).

NHS Future Forum (2012) The NHS's Role in the Public's Health. Available at: http://www.gov.uk/government/uploads/system/uploads/attachment_data/file/216423/dh_132114.pdf (accessed 27 March 2018).

Chapter 4.2: Models of health behaviour

Ajzen, I. (1991) The theory of planned behavior. *Organizational Behavior and Human Decision Processes* 50(2), 179–211.

Becker, M.H. (ed.) (1974) The health belief model and personal health behavior. *Health Education Monographs* 2, 324–473.

Dixon, A. (2008) *Motivation and Confidence: what does it take to change behaviour?* London: Kings Fund.

NICE (2014) Behaviour change. Individual approaches. NICE guideline (PH49). National Institute for Health and Care Excellence. Available at: https://www.nice.org.uk/guidance/ph49 (accessed 27 March 2018).

National Institute for Health and Care Excellence (2007) *Behaviour Change General Approaches Public health guideline (PH6)* NICE: London. https://www.nice.org.uk/guidance/ph6/chapter/2-Considerations (assessed 7 July 2018).

The Behavioural Insights Team (2016) Five factors for supporting people to take a more active role in health and wellbeing. Available at: https://www.behaviouralinsights.co.uk/health/five-factors-for-supporting-people-to-take-a-more-active-role-in-health-and-wellbeing/ (accessed 29 May 2018).

Chapter 4.3: Models and theories of behaviour change

Cialdini, R.B. (2007) *Influence: the Psychology of Persuasion.* New York: Harper Collins.

Prochaska, J.O. and Diclimente, C. (1984) *The Transtheoretical Approach. Crossing Traditional Foundations of Change.* Illinois: Irwin.

Public Health England (2018) Change4Life Campaigns. Overview and Resources. Available at: https://campaignresources.phe.gov.uk/resources/campaigns/17-change4life/overview (accessed 29 May 2018).

Thaler, R.H. and Sunstein, C.R. (2009) *Nudge – Improving Decisions About Health, Wealth and Happiness.* London: Penguin.

Chapter 4.4: Readiness to change

Dalton, C.C. & Gottlieb, L.N. (2003) The concept of readiness to change. *Journal of Advanced Nursing* 42(2): 108–117.

Michie, S., van Stralen, M.M. and West, R. (2011) The behaviour change wheel: A new method for characterising and designing behaviour change interventions. *Implementation Science* 6: 42.

Further reading

Michie, S., Hyder, N., Walia, A. and West, R. (2011) Development of a taxonomy of behaviour change techniques used in individual behavioural support for smoking cessation. *Addictive Behaviours* 36: 315–319.

Chapter 4.5: Self-efficacy and resilience

Antonovsky, A. (1987) *Unravelling the Mystery of Health. How People Manage Stress and Stay Well.* San-Francisco: Jossey Boss.

Bandura, A. (1997) *Self-Efficacy: The Exercise of Control.* New York: Freeman.

Hill, M., Stafford, A., Seaman, P., Ross, N. and Daniel, B. (2007) *Parenting and Resilience – A Literature Review.* York: Joseph Rowntree Foundation.

Pemberton, C. (2015) *Resilience. A Practical Guide for Coaches.* Oxford: OUP.

Reivich, K. and Shatte, A. (2003) *The Resilience Factor. 7 Keys to finding your inner strength and overcoming life's hurdles.* London: Penguin Random House.

Schwarzer, R. and Warner, L.M. (2013) Perceived self-efficacy and its relationship to resilience. In: Prince-Embury, S. and Saklofske, D.H. (eds), *Resilience in Children, Adolescents, and Adults: Translating Research into Practice.* New York: Springer, pp. 139–150.

Chapter 4.6: Skills to support behaviour change

Miller, W.R. and Rollnick, S. (2002) *Motivational Interviewing. Preparing people to change addictive behaviour,* 2nd edn. New York: Guilford Press.

Miller, W.R. and Sanchez, V.C. (1994) Motivating young adults for treatment and lifestyle change. In: Howard, G.S. and Nathan, P.E. (eds), *Alcohol Use and Misuse by Young Adults.* Notre Dame, IN: University of Notre Dame Press, pp. 55–81.

National Institute for Health and Care Excellence (2006) Smoking: brief Interventions and referrals. Manchester: NICE Available at: https://www.nice.org.uk/guidance/ph1?unlid=93832449620162193023 (accessed 29 March 2018).

National Obesity Observatory (2011) Brief interventions for weight management. Available at: https://www.hse.ie/eng/health/child/healthyeating/weightmanagement.pdf (accessed 29 May 2018).

Rollnick, S., Miller, W.R. and Butler, C.C. (2008) *Motivational Interviewing in Health Care. Helping Patients Change Behaviour.* New York: Guildford Press.

Rollnick, S., Butler, C.C., Kinnersley, P., Gregory, J. and Mash, B. (2010) Motivational Interviewing. *British Medical Journal* 340: 1242–1245.

Rosengren, D.B. (2009) *Building Motivational Interviewing Skills. A Practitioner Workbook.* New York: Guilford Press.

World Health Organization (2010) The ASSIST-linked brief intervention for hazardous and harmful substance use. A manual for use in primary care. Geneva: WHO. Available at: http://www.who.int/substance_abuse/publications/assist_sbi/en/ (accessed 29 March 2018).

World Health Organization (2014) Toolkit for delivering the 5A's and 5R's brief tobacco interventions in primary care. Geneva: WHO. Available at: http://www.who.int/tobacco/publications/smoking_cessation/9789241506953/en/ (accessed 29 March 2018).

Chapter 4.7: Skills supporting behaviour change. Example 1: Jenna

Becker, M.H. (1974) *The Health Belief Model and Personal Health Behaviour.* C.B. Slack.

Rosenstock, I.M. (1966) Why people use health services. *Millbank Memorial Fund Quarterly* 44: 94–124.

Chapter 4.8: Skills supporting behaviour change. Example 2: Rachel

Cialdini, R.B. (2007) *Influence: The Psychology of Persuasion*. New York: Harper Collins.

Chapter 5.1: Community health and public health

Blaxter, M. (2007) Evidence for the effect on inequalities in health of interventions designed to change behaviour. Bristol: Department of Social Medicine, University of Bristol. Available at: https://www.nice.org.uk/guidance/ph6/documents/evidence-for-the-effect-on-inequalities-designed-to-change-behaviour2 (accessed 29 March 2018).

Marmot, M. (2010) Fair Society. Healthy Lives. London: UCL Institute of Health Equity. Available at: http://www.instituteofhealthequity.org/resources-reports/fair-society-healthy-lives-the-marmot-review/fair-society-healthy-lives-full-report-pdf.pdf (accessed 29 May 2018).

NICE (2007) Behaviour change: general approaches. National Institute for Health and Care Excellence. Available at: https://www.nice.org.uk/guidance/ph6 (accessed 29 March 2018).

NICE (2016) Community engagement: improving health and wellbeing and reducing health inequalities. National Institute for Health and Care Excellence. Available at: https://www.nice.org.uk/guidance/NG44 (accessed 29 March 2018).

Nuffield Council on Bioethics (2007) Public health: ethical issues. London: Nuffield Council on Bioethics. Available at: http://nuffieldbioethics.org/wp-content/uploads/2014/07/Public-health-ethical-issues.pdf (accessed 29 March 2018).

Rowlingson, K. (2011) Does income inequality cause health and social problems? York: Joseph Rowntree Foundation. Available at: https://www.jrf.org.uk/sites/default/files/jrf/migrated/files/inequality-income-social-problems-full.pdf (accessed 29 March 2018).

Chapter 5.2: Factors that influence the health of communities

Davies, S.C., Winpenny, E., Ball, S., Fowler, T., Rubin, J. and Nolte, E. (2014) For debate: a new wave in public health improvement. *The Lancet* 384, 1889–1895.

Department of Health (2011) Changing Behaviour, Improving Outcomes. Available at: https://www.gov.uk/government/uploads/system/uploads/attachment_data/file/215610/dh_126449.pdf (accessed 21 May 2018).

Chapter 5.3: Barriers to the success of community health improvement programmes

Franks, H., Hardiker, N.R., McGrath, M. and McQuarrie, C. (2012) Public health interventions and behaviour change. Reviewing the grey literature. *Public Health* 126(1), 12–17.

Hardiker, N.R., McGrath, M. and McQuarrie, C. (2009) A synthesis of grey literature around public health interventions and programmes. Salford: University of Salford. Available at: http://usir.salford.ac.uk/12137/1/Public_health_2009.pdf (accessed 21 May 2018).

Chapter 5.4: Factors that may promote the success of community health improvement programmes

Franks, H., Hardiker, N.R., McGrath, M. and McQuarrie, C. (2012) Public health interventions and behaviour change. Reviewing the grey literature. *Public Health* 126(1), 12–17.

Hardiker, N.R., McGrath, M. and McQuarrie, C. (2009) A synthesis of grey literature around public health interventions and programmes. Salford: University of Salford. Available at: http://usir.salford.ac.uk/12137/1/Public_health_2009.pdf (accessed 21 May 2018).

Chapter 6.1: Ethical principles

Beauchamp, T.L. and Childress, J.F. (2009) *Principles of Biomedical Ethics*. Oxford University Press.

Chapter 6.2: Nursing and ethics

NMC (2015) The Code. Professional standards of practice and behaviour for nurses and midwives. Nursing and Midwifery Council.

Peate, I. and Wild, K. (2018) *Nursing Practice. Knowledge and Care*, 2nd edn. Chichester: Wiley-Blackwell.

Chapter 6.3: Application of ethical principles to public health issues

Shaw, D., Macpherson, L. and Conway, D. (2009) Tackling socially determined dental inequalities: ethical aspects of Childsmile, the national oral health demonstration programme in Scotland. *Bioethics* 23(2), 131–139.

Chapter 6.4: The stewardship model

Killoran, A. and White, P. (2010) NICE public health guidance. *Journal of Public Health* 32(1), 136–137.

Nuffield Council on Bioethics (2007) *Public Health: Ethical Issues*. Cambridge: Cambridge Publishers Ltd.

Chapter 6.5: Acceptable health goals

Nuffield Council on Bioethics (2007) *Public Health: Ethical Issues*. Cambridge: Cambridge Publishers Ltd.

Nuffield Council on Bioethics (2010) NICE adopts stewardship model for public health. Available at: http://nuffieldbioethics.org/news/2010/nice-adopts-stewardship-model-for-public-health/ (accessed 21 May 2018).

Chapter 6.6: Opportunity and choice versus coercion

Local Government Association (2013) Changing behaviours in public health – to nudge or to shove? Available at: https://local.gov.uk/sites/default/files/documents/changing-behaviours-publi-e0a.pdf (accessed 22 May 2018).

Chapter 6.7: Individual versus collective interests in public health strategies

Dahlgren, G. and Whitehead, M. (1991) *Policies and Strategies to Promote Social Equity in Health*. Stockholm: Institute for Future Studies.

Department of Health (2010) *Healthy Lives, Healthy People: Our strategy for public health in England*. London: The Stationery Office.

Public Health England (2016) *Strategic Plan for the Next Four Years: Better Outcomes by 2020*. London: PHE.

Chapter 6.8: Individual versus collective interests in public health. Example 1 – Alcohol

NICE (National Institute for Health and Care Excellence) (2011) Alcohol-use disorders: diagnosis, assessment and management of harmful drinking and alcohol dependence. Clinical guideline [CG115]. Available at: https://www.nice.org.uk/guidance/cg115/chapter/introduction (accessed 22 May 2018).

ONS (Office for National Statistics) (2016) Drug use, alcohol and smoking. Available at: https://www.ons.gov.uk/peoplepopulationandcommunity/healthandsocialcare/drugusealcoholandsmoking (accessed 22 May 2018).

Public Health England (2016) *Guidance. Health matters: Harmful drinking and alcohol dependence*. London: PHE.

Chapter 6.9: Individual versus collective issues in public health. Example 2 – People with learning disabilities

DH (2001) *Seeking Consent: Working with People with Learning Disabilities*. London: Department of Health.

Mencap (2007) *Death by Indifference*. London: Mencap.

NMC (2015) *The Code: Professional standards of practice and behaviour for nurses and midwives*. London: Nursing and Midwifery Council.

Peate, I. and Wild, K.(2018) *Nursing Practice: Knowledge and Care*, 2nd edn. Chichester: Wiley Blackwell.

Public Health England (2015) *The Determinants of Health Inequities Experienced by Children with Learning Disabilities*. London: PHE.

Public Health England (2016) *Health and Care of People with Learning Disabilities*. London: PHE.

UK Learning Disability Consultant Nurse Network (2006) *Shaping the Future, A Vision for Learning Disabilities Nursing*. UK Learning Disability Consultant Nurse Network.

Chapter 6.10: Ethical issues in engaging people in conversations about health: an overview

NMC (2015) *The Code. Professional Standards of Practice and Behaviour for Nurses and Midwives*. London: Nursing and Midwifery Council.

Index

Page numbers in **bold** refer to tables or boxes.
Page numbers in *italic* refer to figures.

Public Health and Health Promotion for Nurses at a Glance, First Edition. Karen Wild and Maureen McGrath.
© 2019 John Wiley & Sons Ltd. Published 2019 by John Wiley & Sons Ltd.